STRONG
IS THE NEW
BEAUTIFUL

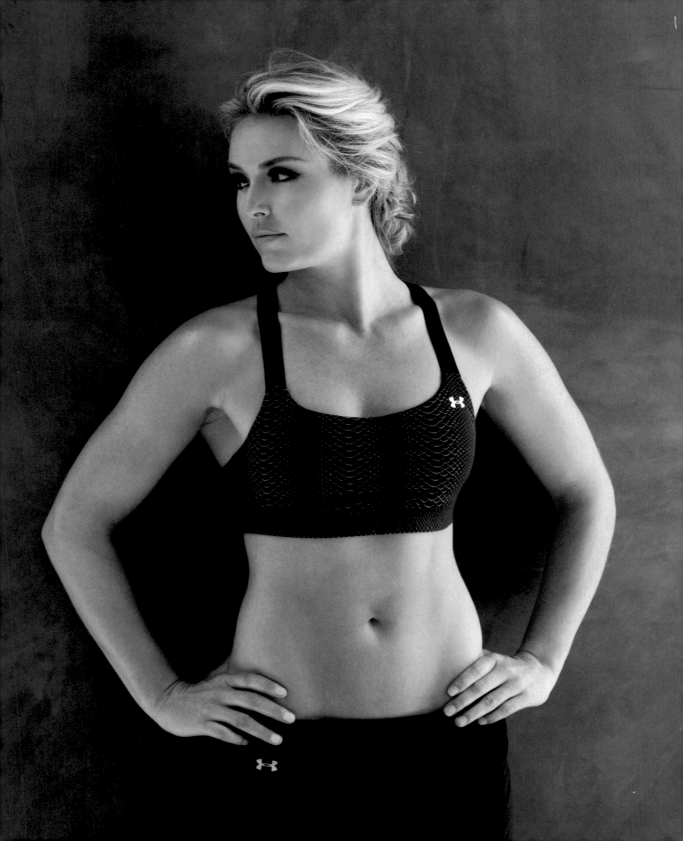

STRONG
IS THE NEW
BEAUTIFUL

Embrace Your Natural Beauty,
Eat Clean, and Harness Your Power

—

Lindsey Vonn
AND SARAH TOLAND

DEY ST.
An Imprint of WILLIAM MORROW

DEY ST.

This book is written as a source of information only. The information contained in this book should by no means be considered a substitute for the advice of a qualified medical professional, who should always be consulted before beginning any new diet, exercise or other health program.

All efforts have been made to ensure the accuracy of the information contained in this book as of the date published. The author and the publisher expressly disclaim responsibility for any adverse effects arising from the use or application of the information contained herein or for any injuries suffered or damages or losses incurred as a result of following the exercise program in this book. All of the procedures, poses, and postures should be carefully studied and clearly understood before attempting them at home.

FIRST EDITION

Designed by Ashley Tucker
All photography by Lauren Ross except the following:
Photograph on page vii © by Chris Fanning
Photographs on pages 4–23, courtesy of the author
Photographs on pages 165–229 © by Jesse Starr, JesseStarrProductions.com

Library of Congress Cataloging-in-Publication Data has been applied for.

ISBN 978-0-06-240058-1 (hardcover)
ISBN 978-0-06-266303-0 (Barnes & Noble signed edition)
ISBN 978-0-06-266301-6 (Target signed edition)

16 17 18 19 20 ov/QGT 10 9 8 7 6 5 4 3 2 1

To those who don't think
they are beautiful enough.
You are beautiful no
matter what size you are.

“ When you commit to getting strong, you agree to go on an incredible journey that will transform you. **”**

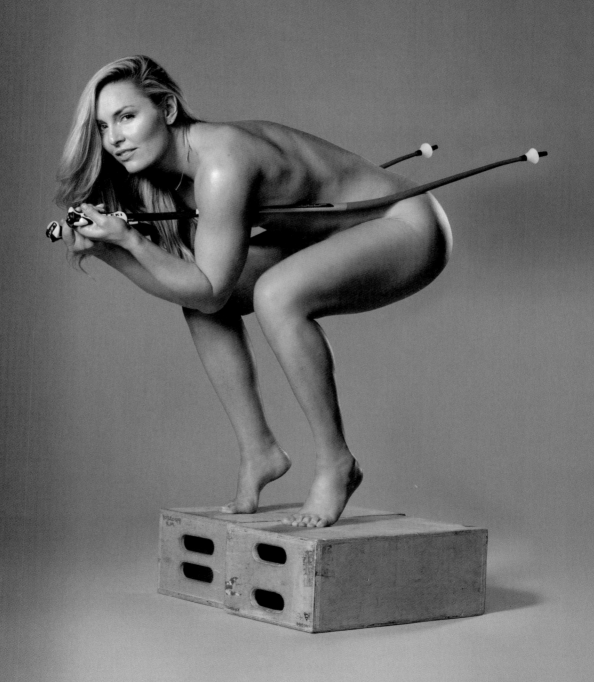

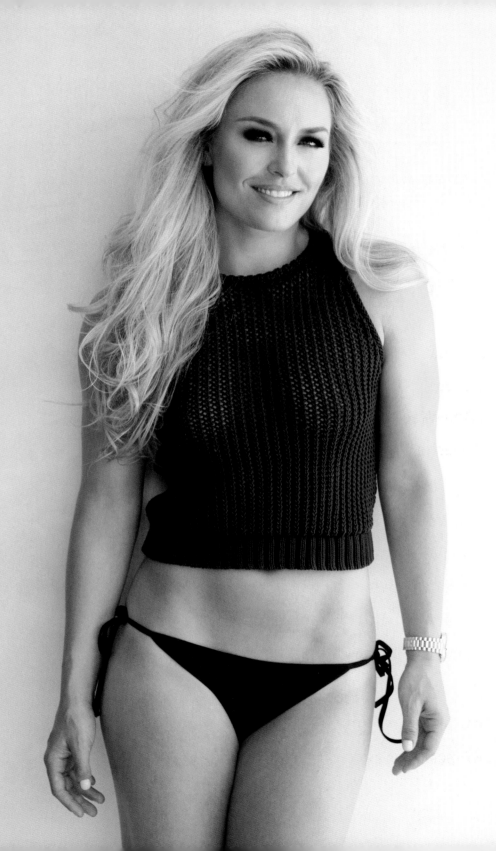

CONTENTS

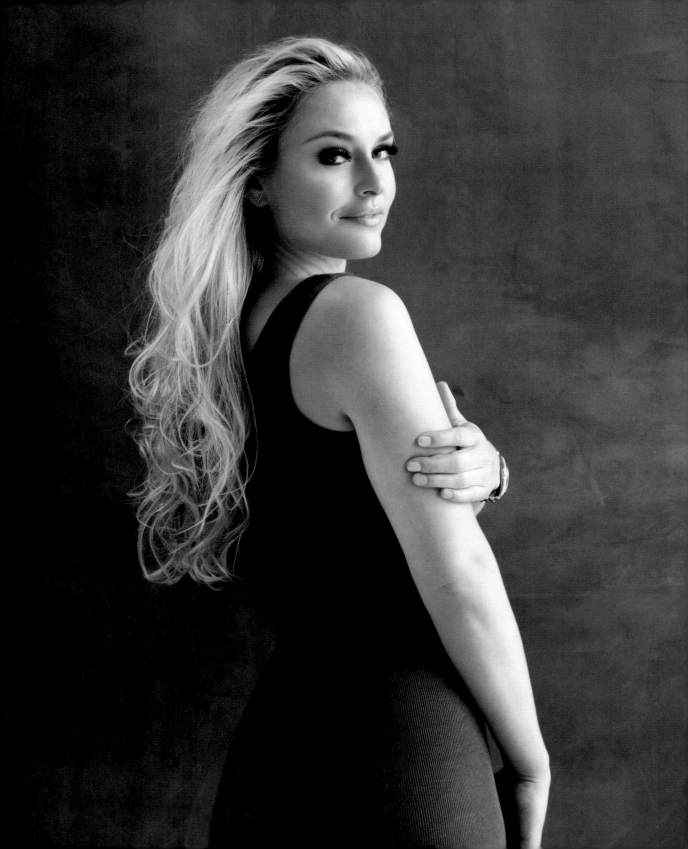

MY LIFE IS MY (STRONG) BODY

One of the most beautiful places I've ever skied is Cortina, Italy. When you're at the top of the mountain where the World Cup is held, all you can see in every direction are peaks and sky, the steep edges of the Dolomites ringing the summit view as if the valleys below don't even exist. Up there, you are closer to the stratosphere than you are to the earth, but there the earth is too, below you and all around you, pushing up rock and jagged snowy hills that seem so unconquerable—unconquerable to everyone but you, standing there on the top of the mountain with the world laid out before you.

That is where I stood—and how I felt—the morning after I tied the all-time record for the most World Cup wins ever by a female skier. It was daybreak, and the sky had blanched to a powdery blue, with just a few sun-rimmed clouds washing through the peaks and coloring the snow below a shimmery gold. I still had to race that day and I was on the hill so early to inspect the course, but I wasn't concerned about the competition ahead. Instead, all I could think about was what I had just accomplished—tying a world record, something I had never thought possible—and all I had endured to stand at that place at that point in time. I was immensely relieved and proud, but most of all, I felt strong, physically and mentally, like I could do anything with my body and mind that I put my heart to.

I hadn't always felt this way, though—so strong, so unstoppable, so on top of the world in more ways than one. Over the course of my career, there had been days, weeks, even months when I felt low, unsure of myself, worried about whether I would ski again, and even worried whether I was too muscular and big to fit into some American ideal of an athlete. I never doubted my ability per se, but getting strong and fit and feeling as good about my body as possible required a journey of sorts. But standing on my skis in Cortina on January 19, 2015—the same day I would go on to not just tie but break the all-time record for most World Cup wins ever—I knew it was a journey that had changed my life and body indelibly, for the better.

I wanted to write this book to share with you my journey and give you the inspiration, tips, and tools you need to change your life and body, too. No matter who you are, what you do for your living, or what your body looks like now, you can get stronger, leaner, healthier, and happier, just as I have. I'm not a coach, trainer, or nutritionist, but I am an Olympic athlete who's tried nearly every exercise and diet there is, and I know what works and what doesn't.

What I've learned, too, is that there's more than one way of exercising and eating that can make you feel good about yourself and your body—and having more than one option is a fabulous thing. While plenty of diet and fitness "experts" will recommend only one way to eat or work out to lose weight or get healthy, I find restrictions to be extremely limiting. We all have different bodies, genetics, preferences, and lifestyles, and I believe that if you want to look and feel your best, you need options that will empower you, not rules that will make exercising and healthy eating that much more difficult.

Since I was young, my life has been about my body, as I've spent nearly all of the past three decades managing my energy, working on my strength, eating and exercising for optimal performance, and preventing and rehabbing the injuries that are as much a part of skiing as the cold and the snow. I'm constantly assessing how I feel, how my muscles look and respond, what exactly is going on in my body, and whether I'm eating the best foods and doing the most effective workouts I can to get to the top step of the Olympic podium.

What I've learned along the way is that no matter what kind of body type you have, making it your goal to get strong rather than to lose a bunch of weight, reach a certain number on the scale, or simply get skinny is a healthier, more sustainable, and ultimately more effective way to change your body—and change it for good. When you make your goal to get strong, you're setting an intention to help your body become fitter and healthier, not just smaller or thinner. You agree to try new ways of eating and exercising that you can sustain for life—not just for a few weeks or months—as you find those foods and workouts that you actually enjoy, not just the ones you eat or suffer through because you want to lose weight. When you work to get strong, you also agree to get mentally fit, building up your confidence in and out of the gym as you feel better about yourself. You stop doing the workouts you don't like, you stop eating too little or those foods that don't taste good, and you stop the body shaming, as you focus on feeling good about what you eat, how you exercise, and how you look and feel. Because getting strong doesn't mean just getting lean, but trying to find personal purpose and empowerment, too. Because when you're strong, you too can do anything you set your mind, body, and heart to. Trust me . . . I know.

My journey to get strong started when I was a teenager, although my quest to be an athlete began when I was much younger. The oldest of five, I was born in Burnsville, Minnesota, a suburb outside the Twin Cities. By no stretch of the imagination could Burnsville be considered a ski town. We had just one hill, Buck Hill, with a 310-foot vertical drop—shorter than most waterslides.

But Buck Hill was only five minutes from my family's home, and my father, Alan, a former ski racer and junior national ski champion, was a ski coach there. When I was just a baby, he took me out in a backpack on the hill, and before I was three, I was learning to take my first turns on skis.

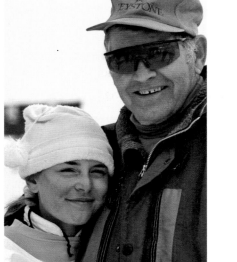

With my Grandpa Don at the Junior Olympics.

I always enjoyed skiing more than the other sports I tried as a kid—soccer, gymnastics, ice-skating, running, and the other activities that most children try in grade school. Nothing made me happier than being on a mountain, especially when I was racing down one as fast as I could. I wasn't particularly quick on skis when I was young—quite the opposite, in fact—but I always looked forward to my time on the mountain. It was fun being outside in the snow, carving down the hill run after run, first with my father, then with my friends. When it got too cold to ski anymore, I'd huddle inside the lodge with hot chocolate and doughnuts, and to me, the sport was much more special than any soccer game.

By the time I was seven, I knew that I wanted to race. I joined the Buck Hill team, which was led at the time by Erich Sailer, the first development coach ever to be inducted into the U.S. Ski and Snowboard Hall of Fame—he was also my father's coach when my dad was a racer. I wasn't fast, and I can remember Erich chiding my father that he had produced a turtle of a daughter on the hill.

That I was slow only fueled my determination to get faster, and when I was nine, I convinced my parents to let me travel alone to a ski camp in Austria. I was the youngest camper there by several years, but my age didn't bother me. My dad had given me an envelope full of different kinds of foreign currency—Austrian schillings, German marks—and I felt incredibly grown up and independent. Plus, I was skiing with kids who were so much older and better than me, and I had no choice but to keep up or get left behind. All in all, the experience was just what I needed to boost my confidence in myself and my skiing. It was also my first exposure to speaking German—or rather, not being able to speak it—and after returning home, I immediately decided to start learning the language.

Several months later, something incredible happened. At the local ski shop down the road from my family's home, I met Picabo Street, who at that time was the most successful American female skier. I had posters of Picabo plastered on my bedroom wall, and when I finally met her in person, it was like seeing a superhero—I couldn't believe she was real. I had never met a professional ski racer

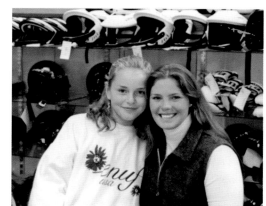

Meeting Picabo Street.

before or even really knew that skiing could be something you could do as a full-time career. Yet there was Picabo, a woman who had made a life out of skiing, and I thought to myself, *I want to do that, too.*

Afterward, I took my racing more seriously. I spoke with my father, and we realized together that if I wanted to get better, I would need to start skiing in the mountains, not just on little Buck Hill. I began making trips to Vail, Colorado, for training camps, mostly with my mother at first, but as I got faster and faster and started to show real potential, eventually my whole family, including my four siblings—my sister Karin and the triplets, Reed, Dylan, and Laura—all moved to Vail with me.

I was only thirteen at the time, but I was old enough to know that my family was making a giant sacrifice, all for my skiing career. To move to Vail, my parents had to sell the house they'd built in Burnsville, which had been their dream home, and my brothers and sisters had to leave their friends and everything familiar to go to new schools and make new friends. This put a tremendous amount of pressure on me and made me that much more resolute in my training—because there was no way I was going to let my family down.

One of the earliest indicators that I would make it as a pro skier occurred the year after we moved to Vail, when I won the juniors competition at Trofeo Topolino in Italy. I was just fourteen, but the victory made me the first American female ever to win the title. Every skier who'd won Topolino before had gone on to win a World Cup—the premier event in alpine skiing, part of a large international circuit. Standing on the Topolino podium in Italy, thousands of miles from Vail, I finally felt that whatever turtle Erich Sailer had seen at Buck Hill was long gone and that I was at last headed in the right direction.

My next step was to make the U.S. Ski Team, which required passing a physical fitness test. I joined my parents' gym and began strength training. My father also started me on a regimen of doing 100 push-ups and 100 sit-ups every night, and took me to the track on the weekends to run.

I hated running; in fact, I loathed it (and I still do). When I ran, everything hurt: my knees, shins, quads. At that time I didn't like lifting weights either, but I did both regularly and religiously, and when I was fifteen, the work paid off: I made the team's developmental program.

Once on the team, I knew my physical training was just beginning. The team had a sponsorship agreement with a cycling company, which allowed me to get a nice road bike for little money, and I started riding instead of running. Cycling was a big boon to my ability to get fit: I loved it, which meant I was able to do more aerobic exercise more often, with more energy and enjoyment. When I was in Minnesota, where my family moved back to after I made the team, I would ride for miles on long, scenic farm roads to neighboring towns. In Colorado, I started biking up Vail Pass, which was challenging, but so much more exciting—and rewarding—than running an arbitrary number of miles around a track.

As I got stronger and stronger off skis, I became faster and faster on the hill, and my status on the team quickly progressed from developmental to C, then B, then A Team, or the top tier of alpine racers in the country. At age sixteen, just one year after earning a berth on the team, I raced my first World Cup in Park City, Utah,

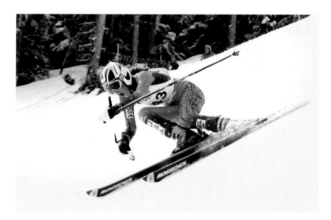

Racing at Whistler.

and then picked up my first official World Cup points shortly after in Val d'Isère, France, in what would become a very familiar race for me over the next fifteen years.

In 2002, my life changed in an extraordinary way: I made the U.S.

Olympic team. I could hardly believe that the girl from Buck Hill would now be an Olympic athlete—a term that carried so much weight in the world and one that I had only dreamed about for years, like so many other aspiring skiers. Once I was at the Games, it almost didn't matter to me how well I raced—simply making the team was a success in itself. At the opening ceremony in Salt Lake, I remember walking into the stadium and letting the roar of the crowd wash over me. Lost in the noise and the emotion of the moment, I started to feel a huge sense of relief welling up inside of me as I realized that the sacrifices my family had made were paying off in a very real, qualitative way. Days later, I placed sixth in the combined event, the best result from the U.S. women's team at the Games that year.

After the Olympics, I continued to improve in small, measured ways, but I wasn't progressing as quickly as I had before. I knew I could be doing more to get my body stronger, and at my dad's recommendation, I used two years of a paid advance against my potential earnings to hire my first real coach, a Polish trainer named Jacques Choynowski who had helped transform other elite skiers in the past.

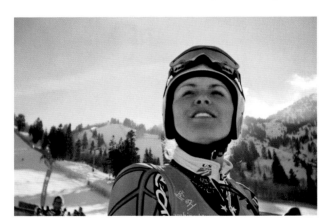

At the 2002 Olympics.

Jacques lived in Monaco in a tiny one-bedroom apartment with his girlfriend, so at age nineteen I moved to Monaco for the summer to train. It was an intense situation in many ways, but I worked out harder in Monaco with Jacques than I ever had before in my life. For the most part, he was an old-school coach, the kind who thought you should push yourself until you puked, which I nearly did after every workout.

The following season, 2004–2005, I made the podium, placing in the top three, at my first World Cup race in Cortina, Italy. In many ways, this was a bigger accomplishment than making the Olympic team, because it meant that I was no longer simply *on* the World Cup circuit, but I was a contender there, too. It was also a big confidence boost, and one that gave me the push I needed to aim higher. At the beginning of the following season, I won my first World Cup in Lake Louise, Canada, and finished the year with five more podiums.

That winter I was spending more time with my boyfriend, who was also on the U.S. team, and I moved from Vail to Park City, where he and the rest of the team trained. I also started doing their regular workouts and following a high-carb diet, which the team nutritionist recommended and which was popular at the time with many endurance athletes.

It didn't take more than a few months of eating mostly pasta, cereal, and bagels for me to start feeling tired and lethargic, as if I were getting heavier, not more muscular or faster. It bothered me too that when I stood in front of the mirror in the gym, I didn't think that my body looked very athletic, even though I was working out up to six hours a day. Eventually, I didn't feel I could maintain that kind of training or diet anymore, and I decided to start working with Picabo Street's old trainer, Matt James.

Matt helped revitalize my workouts, giving my training the structure and boost it needed. Soon I started to see the same kind of gains in my strength and racing that I had after spending time with Jacques in Monaco. I was getting stronger and skiing faster, and even though I still didn't necessarily like how my body looked in the mirror all the time, I could tell visually that I was adding the muscle I wanted.

While I was with Matt, my skiing got another big boost: I got sponsored by Red Bull after many interviews with the company. This was a major advancement for my career. The energy drink maker is an icon in American sports; more important, being asked to join signified that I had made it as professional skier. Moreover, Red Bull had sponsored only two or three other skiers in its entire history, and I felt special and honored to be asked to join.

After signing with Red Bull, I started working with the company's coach, Martin Hager. Martin's training was completely different from anything I had experienced before. I started spending more time on the bike, which was exhilarating, and seeing a physical therapist, getting regular massages, and experimenting more with what I ate and when. As I got stronger, I finally started to look like the toned athlete I hoped to be. Finally, the ways I was training and eating were paying off in positive, tangible ways. I went to Austria with Martin to train, and Red Bull hired a language coach to help me work on my German. Once again, I felt like everything was coming together.

But no amount of training or confidence at the time could have prepared me for what is nearly inevitable in skiing: falls. Of all times, at all places, my first debilitating crash occurred during the 2006 Olympics in Italy. I caught an edge, my legs split, and I launched off a jump backward, landing on my back. For a few moments, I couldn't move, and the feeling of paralysis suspended all my senses—I couldn't believe what was happening to me. For the first time in what would become several occasions, I had to be airlifted off the mountain. I panicked, and during that awful helicopter ride to the hospital, all I could think was that I had broken my back and that I'd never ski again, all at the age of twenty-one. When I had started training that day, I had been on top of the world, about to compete in my second Olympics, daydreaming of a medal after a string of World Cup wins. Now, moments later, I was strapped onto a stretcher, a thousand feet in the air, being moved noisily away from what I believed would be the last mountain I would ever ski.

After I was rushed into the hospital, the doctors ordered a series of MRIs and CT scans before they delivered the news: I was going to be okay. It was only some bad bruising, and I would be in a lot of pain, but nothing was broken, and I would ski again. I was relieved, overwhelmed, and thankful—and then anxious to get back to the Games. The pain was intense, but I gritted my teeth and raced through it, finishing eighth in the downhill and seventh in the super G. I was disappointed that I hadn't finished stronger, but I was more grateful than anything just to be able to ski. Plus, I had learned one of the most important lessons of my life: Never take skiing for granted.

The following season, I doubled down on my training with Martin, increasing the amount of time I spent in the gym and focusing more energy on getting stronger, not only so that I could ski faster but also so that my body could better handle crashes like the one I had just endured. Once again, the grueling training paid off: At the 2007 World Championships that winter, I medaled for the first time, taking home silver in both the downhill and the super G.

That fall, Thomas and I were married in Deer Valley, Utah. I was in love, felt fabulous about my life and career, and not surprisingly went on to have a triumphant season that year, winning both the downhill and the overall World Cup title for the first time.

But I still hadn't won gold on the world's biggest stage yet: the World Championships, which has the same depth and level of competition as the Olympics. This bothered me, especially since there had been speculation in the press that I couldn't win gold when it really mattered—at large international championships such as the World Champs or the

Olympics, when the pressure was high. I knew in my heart this wasn't true, but I still had to prove it to myself. I started training even harder on and off the hill for the next World Champs, which would be held in Val d'Isère, where I had earned my first World Cup points.

Still, for as much speed and power as I could gain, I knew I needed a different kind of strength if I wanted to win a world championship: mental strength. As my career had progressed, the expectation that I would win had increased. At previous World Champs, I had tried to handle this mounting pressure by either being too relaxed or too aggressive. Neither approach had worked well for me, and right before Val d'Isère, I realized why: Being too relaxed left me racing without the grit I needed, while being too aggressive meant I couldn't relax and let my body and mind do what they needed to do—and had done so often in training—to win. Somehow I had to learn how to combine the two approaches, to find my own sense of calm while keeping the aggressive edge I needed. With this new attitude, I went to Val d'Isère feeling mentally prepared for the first time, and not only did I get the gold I wanted, I got two of them—one in the downhill and one in the super G.

Knowing that I could win when the pressure was high was precisely the confidence boost I needed before the 2009-2010 season—the same year as the Winter Olympics in Vancouver. With two gold medals now from the World Champs, I felt that I had a good chance to repeat the feat and grab the biggest gold of all time—one from the Olympic Games. I also felt stronger than I had in years, and soon after the season started, I began to rack up wins on the World Cup circuit, surpassing Bode Miller to become the American skier with the most World Cup wins ever.

I was so physically and mentally focused on the 2010 Olympics that I didn't think anything could deter me from getting what I wanted. But I was wrong. Two weeks before the Vancouver Games, I crashed during a training run. I didn't have to be medevacked off the mountain, but I had a badly bruised shin. I couldn't ski at all and wouldn't be able to until the games.

Suddenly I found myself in the eye of what appeared to be the perfect storm: I was on the cover of *Sports Illustrated* that month, and I knew that everyone in the States expected me to medal. Some had even speculated that I could win as many as five gold medals. The pressure on me was higher than it had ever been before, yet I couldn't even ski and was in excruciating pain just walking. I wouldn't even think of backing out, but how could I medal if I couldn't make it down the hill?

Not taking myself too seriously helps balance the moments of pressure.

I knew that I had to do something to take myself out of the center of the storm. After flying to Vancouver and doing the usual media rounds, I holed up in a condo that Red Bull had rented for me. It was a difficult decision to make, but I also told the team that I wasn't going to participate in the opening ceremony that year, and I didn't even watch it on TV. In fact, I forced myself not to watch any of the Olympic coverage, even though I knew some of it inevitably included speculation about me. I told my friends that I couldn't see them until after my events, spending time only with my sister and brother, both of whom helped me stay calm, and I deliberately shut down all my social media. In a stroke of good luck, the figurative storm I felt around me turned into a literal storm, causing rain for days, which delayed my race date, giving my shin more time to recover.

Finally it was time to race. I knew that I was as ready as I'd ever be, even though I hadn't been able to train to capacity the last few weeks and my shin was still sore. I told myself that all I could do was my best, whatever that was, and with this attitude, in my first race of the games, in the downhill, I had the best moment of my life and career to date: I won an Olympic gold medal.

Exhausted and jubilant at the bottom of the course, when I realized that I had won, I was so overcome with emotion that I couldn't speak when a reporter asked me what it felt like to be an Olympic champion. All I could think about was everything that my family had given up, everything that I had given up until that point in my life, and how it was all worth it for that single moment. I cried with relief and joy, both through the interview and during the awards ceremony afterward. When I won

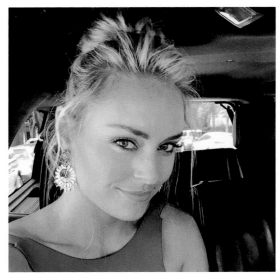

Red carpet ready!

a bronze medal in the super G days later, it was just the sweet completion to the experience—it would take weeks, if not months, for it to sink in that I was a two-time Olympic medalist. And while others might have expected me to podium in every discipline, five Olympic medals had never been my goal. I had two, and one was gold, and I was immensely proud and grateful.

When I returned home after the Olympics, my life suddenly changed: I was a celebrity. I had been skiing, winning races, and breaking records for years, but being an Olympic champion seemed to switch on some kind of spotlight that instantly illuminated me as an athlete in the eyes of many Americans. Like other Olympic champions, I began to be invited to Hollywood events, movie premieres, and parties. People on the street recognized me, and producers started calling to book me on morning and late-night TV shows.

All the attention surprised me at first, and in the beginning, I loved getting dressed up, walking the red carpet, and meeting famous people I had seen only on-screen. But the more time I spent at these events, the more I began to feel that I didn't quite fit in. I was taller than most of the women, and even many of the men, but I also felt bigger and much more muscular. When I looked around, it seemed like everyone was model-thin, with tiny waists and long, willowy legs, all of them so small, compact, and stereotypically beautiful— So unlike me, I thought.

Before the Olympics, I had been immersed in my own aesthetic world, the world of skiing, where everyone looks like I do. My female competitors were just as muscular as I was, as were most of the elite female athletes from other sports whom I'd met. But now I was in a realm where being skinny seemed to matter more than being healthy—and certainly more than being fit. I started to question myself. As I stared at my body in the mirror, I thought: *Should I not wear this dress? Do I need to lose weight if I want to stay socially relevant as an athlete?*

These insecurities haunted me into the following season, and I became more concerned with how I looked in the mirror than with how strong I felt in the gym or on the hill. Winning an Olympic gold had also softened some of my drive, which detracted from my training, too. I knew I wasn't pushing myself as hard, not giving it my all during every training run or trying to lift every ounce of weight that I could. I felt directionless for almost the whole season, even as I continued to win World Cup races.

At the end of the year, I missed the overall World Championship title by just three points. It was such a narrow and disappointing defeat that it shook me. I knew that I was hurting my career, and for what? My perception of someone else's perception of what was beautiful? I was an Olympic athlete, after all, and Olympic athletes were muscular. I resolved to start training as hard as ever during the following year.

Once again, though, life had a different plan for me, and several weeks into my 2011–2012 season, Thomas and I announced we were getting divorced after almost ten years together. As a result, that fall and winter were difficult and emotional for me because not only had Thomas been my husband, but he had also been my part-time coach, full-time travel companion, advisor, and best friend—in other words, my rock.

Given how much I was struggling emotionally, I knew that I needed to bury myself in my sport that much more. Through all the years and varying ups and downs, skiing was one thing I could rely on to give me a sense of joy in times of hardship. That season, I looked to my training and racing more than I ever had. I kept to myself and focused everything on my career.

At the same time, newspaper articles began to surface questioning whether I could make it as an athlete without a man by my side, as first my father had guided my career, then Thomas. I knew without a doubt that there wasn't any truth in the rumors, but the speculation infuriated me. That season I made it my mission to prove everyone wrong, and unlike most of my competitors, I started planning all my own travel, driving myself to races, and doing all the other things a sports agent, personal assistant, parent, or partner might do. But I discovered that I liked being in charge of my career, and I found the change empowering. I felt more capable, competent, and independent, and even stronger than I had in previous seasons.

Fueled by this newfound strength, I went on that season to break the all-time record for the most points ever scored on the World Cup circuit in a single year. I knew that I was back to being me—physically, mentally, and emotionally. That spring, I met Tiger Woods, and we started dating the following winter.

The following season, 2012-2013, had all the hallmarks to be successful: I felt physically and mentally strong, I was confident, my training was going well, and my life was in a new and exciting place. But early into the World Cup circuit, while racing in Europe, I contracted a serious stomach illness that sent me to the hospital for several days. I couldn't eat much and was consistently low on fluids, and I lost weight, as well as muscle mass, strength, and training time during a critical period. Once out of the hospital, I surprised myself by winning several races in a row, but by the time the holidays came around, I felt weak again, as if I couldn't overcome the energy and muscle loss from earlier in the season.

That was how I felt going into the 2013 World Championships in Austria, yet I was determined to medal and thought I had a good chance. But during the super G, I landed a jump, got stuck into some soft snow and my legs buckled, sending me head over heels down the mountain several times before coming to a hard stop. I could feel right away that something terrible had happened. I began screaming on the side of the hill, I was in so much pain. It was more pain than I had ever felt in my life, and while I was being airlifted off the hill, I was full of anxiety and crying hysterically, thinking that this time my career was finally over.

When the doctors showed me my MRIs at the hospital, I knew right away that my season, if not my career, was finished. I had torn the ACL and MCL in my right knee and fractured my right tibial plateau—the bone near the knee that is one of the most critical weight-bearing bones in the body. What this meant was that my right knee, on which half of my athletic career literally depended, was nearly destroyed—and the 2014 Olympics were only one year away. I was devastated. As soon as I could leave the hospital in Austria, I flew back to Colorado, making fast arrangements to have reconstructive surgery the day after I landed.

Since I had ripped more than one ligament in my knee and fractured a nearby bone, the surgery was long and complicated—so was the recovery process. My right leg looked like some sort of science experiment—swollen, bruised, and crisscrossed with scars—and I was on crutches for weeks. It took a good deal of mental and emotional resolve to remain positive and focus on walking again, let alone training.

Still, the day after I had surgery, with the Olympics in mind, I started doing core work on the therapy table, twisting with a medicine ball and crunching up with weights. Doing something—anything—for my body made me feel instantly better, and as soon as I could be up on crutches, I starting training with my one good leg on a rowing machine and stationary bike with my brace out in front of me. That spring I also started spending more time with Tiger, and being around him helped: He was also a professional athlete, after all, and had undergone similar career-threatening surgeries, and I found it soothing to have someone of his caliber understand what I was going through.

More than half a year after my fall, after months on crutches and doing daily rehab, it was time to test my knee on skis. I flew to Chile, and after I took my first turn, I was instantly relieved: I could ski. I was going to be okay.

In November, I started training with my usual fervor, trying to build up my strength as quickly as possible for the start of 2013-2014 season, which was just one month away. I had missed so much training time, and I knew that I had a long road before me just to catch up to the place where many of my competitors were. With this thought in the back of my mind, I started to treat my workouts as if they were races, flying down training runs at the same speeds I would if I were competing.

It was during one of these agressive runs on Copper Mountain in Colorado, in mid-November, just three months before the Olympic Games, when I crashed again. The fall wasn't as bad as some of my previous ones, but the results were still disastrous: I had retorn the ACL in my right knee.

I was devastated. I felt as if I had worked too long and too hard after my surgery to let something, anything, sideline me. So nine days after my fall, I decided to continue racing with a torn ACL and flew to the World Cup in Lake Louise, Canada. Racing was painful and I felt unsteady, but the fact that I was able to compete gave me hope that I could strengthen the muscles around the ligament enough to be able to race the Games in February.

That December, I returned to Val d'Isère—the course I knew so well—to race the World Cup. But on the downhill, as Tiger watched from the sidelines, I felt my knee suddenly buckle under me, and I pulled up. It was an awful feeling, to have no control over one leg, and I knew that I couldn't keep racing. So I stopped, mid-course—I knew I had reinjured my knee. I flew home and immediately had MRIs. The results weren't good: I had shredded my meniscus. A few weeks later, in mid-January, I announced that I wouldn't compete in the 2014 Olympics.

That winter I sank into depression, something I had battled off and on in the past. I had decided to have my second knee surgery in Florida, but it wasn't close to where Tiger lived, and I also knew he had a busy competition schedule that didn't leave him much time at home. I felt like I needed a friend to help me through yet another long, grueling recovery process—my second in less than a year—and I decided on a whim to drive to a nearby animal shelter. There were so many dogs there, all of

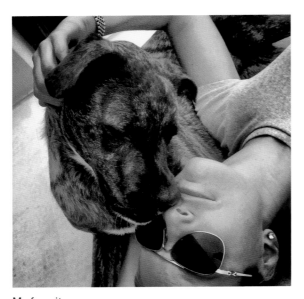

My favorite
roommate:
my dog, Leo.

them barking wildly. Finally I came to the last kennel, where a brindle mutt sat quietly, staring up at me. I asked the shelter workers if I could play with him, and they told that he had recently been hit by a car, had a bad knee, and couldn't be very active. *That makes two of us, buddy*, I thought, and I told them that I wanted Leo, which is what they had already named him.

In late January, Leo, my sister Laura, and I rented a little apartment in Pensacola, near where I had my second surgery. During the operation, while repairing the ACL, they found my meniscus so shredded that they almost had to remove it completely. Thankfully, Dr. Andrews was able to put it back together. Later, I learned that Dr. Andrews had told my trainers that because of all the damage there was only a fifty-fifty chance I'd be able to compete again.

That winter and spring I suffered many dark days as I wrestled with my current reality and my chances of making it back to the top of my sport. My recovery was longer and more involved than that after my first surgery, and I felt defeated whenever I thought about how hard I had worked the year before only to be in the same place, at the same time, all over again. I fought to stay hopeful, but I often didn't feel positive. I had a hard time sleeping, but I didn't want to get up in the morning, either, and there were many days when my physical therapist, Lindsay Winninger, had to pull me out from under the covers.

The physical part was just as draining as the emotional. During my first recovery, I had found strength and resilience in doing physical rehab, but this time around, the exercises felt exhausting and repetitive of everything I had done the year before. It was emotionally difficult to find the will to train, and it was also physically exhausting: I had lost so much muscle in my right leg that it barely seemed to function, making the rehab a continual struggle, day after day.

During that time, there were days when I could see the light at the end of the tunnel, yet more often than not, everything looked black, and I shut down, keeping to myself in my bedroom with only Leo for company. The possibility of skiing again was the only thing that kept me going. This time I didn't care about the competition, the World Cup wins, or the Olympics—I just wanted to be back on the mountain, doing what I love.

Finally, in October, I was ready to try to ski. I took my first turns on my new knee in Saas-Fee, Switzerland, and I knew right away that I had defied the odds again. At the time, I had never been happier to be back on the hill.

That December, I raced my first World Cup in Lake Louise, Canada, where I finished eighth—my worst standing there since 2007. I was angry, only because I knew I could have done so much better, and the disappointment seemed to snap a competitive part of my brain back into place. As a result, the next day I raced the downhill and won, marking my sixtieth World Cup win. Once again, I was back.

That race also meant something else: I was only two victories away from tying Annemarie Moser-Pröll's thirty-five-year-old record of sixty-two World Cup wins. I knew that I didn't have a ton of training under my belt that season, but I believed in myself and thought that I could break the record that winter. Several weeks after Lake Louise, I won the downhill at Val d'Isère, and then tied Moser-Pröll's record in Cortina, Italy.

The day that I broke the record, January 19, 2015, after standing on the Cortina peak that morning, I felt triumphant. My parents, stepparents, sister Laura, and Tiger had all flown to Europe to watch me race, and even though I hadn't been able to go to the 2014 Olympics, after two almost-career-ending surgeries, becoming the most successful female skier ever, to me, was just as good as another Olympic gold.

That season I finished the year with eight World Cup wins and two World Cup titles, tying the all-time world record for a total of nineteen titles. If there had been any question about whether I could come back after double knee surgery, the doubts were over. I was back and on top again.

Something else joyful happened to me that winter: I got Bear. Earlier in the year, I had realized that Leo needed a companion, especially

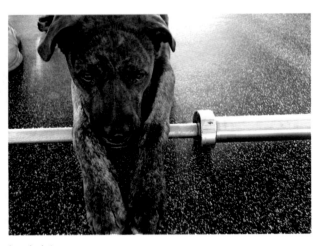

Leo helping me in the gym.

after I began traveling to Europe to ski (and he started hiding in my closet, sad that I was no longer around all the time). So I searched online and found an adorable-looking mutt at a foster home near Vail. Leo and I drove to meet him, and we both fell in love. I called him Bear and took him home.

Several months later, Tiger and I decided to separate. Our relationship had become increasingly difficult to maintain, given our conflicting event schedules and two different homes across the country, and while we parted amicably, I was grateful to have both dogs with me that spring to keep me company and help me through the separation.

———

All in all, it's been nearly thirty years since I started skiing, and my body has accomplished many amazing things. When I look back on life so far, I sometimes can't believe how many hours I've spent in the gym or on the bike, or how many training runs I've done in the snow, rain, blazing sun, or freezing cold. I've raced all over the world and traveled to more countries in one week than many people see in a lifetime. I've tied and broken records and won titles, medals, trophies, crystal globes, even a baby cow. My body has survived horrific crashes, broken bones, torn ligaments, fractured body parts, debilitating pain, and two intense knee surgeries. I've also endured what so many other women have, too: breakups, relationship problems, and a divorce, along with all the insecurities about how my body looks to others and how it looks to me. But I've been fortunate to come through it all, and in the end, I owe everything to my body. My *strong* body.

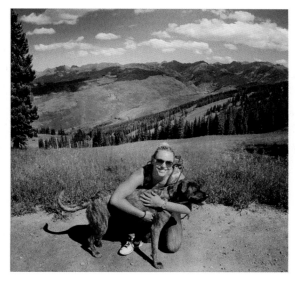

My happy place.

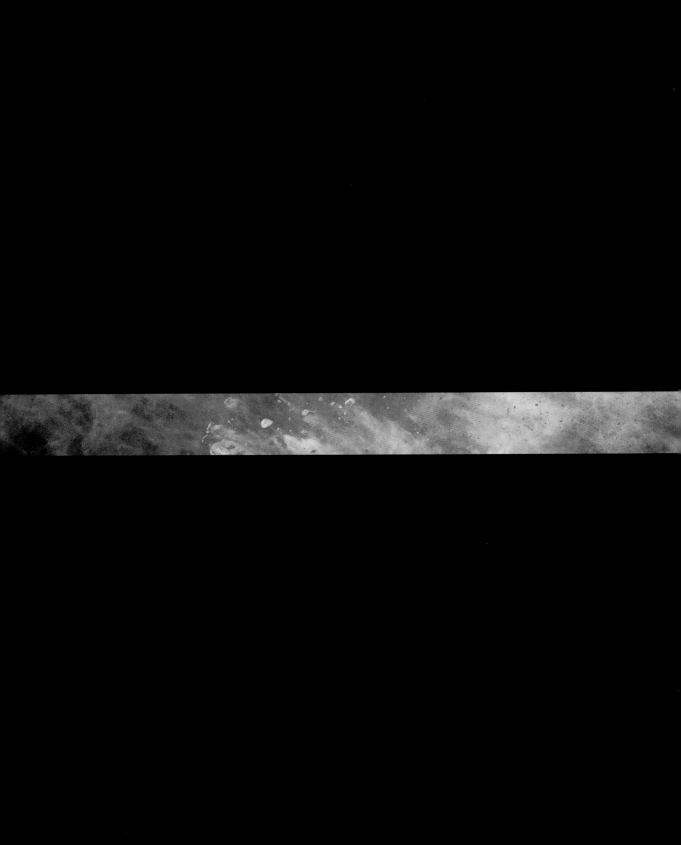

MIND

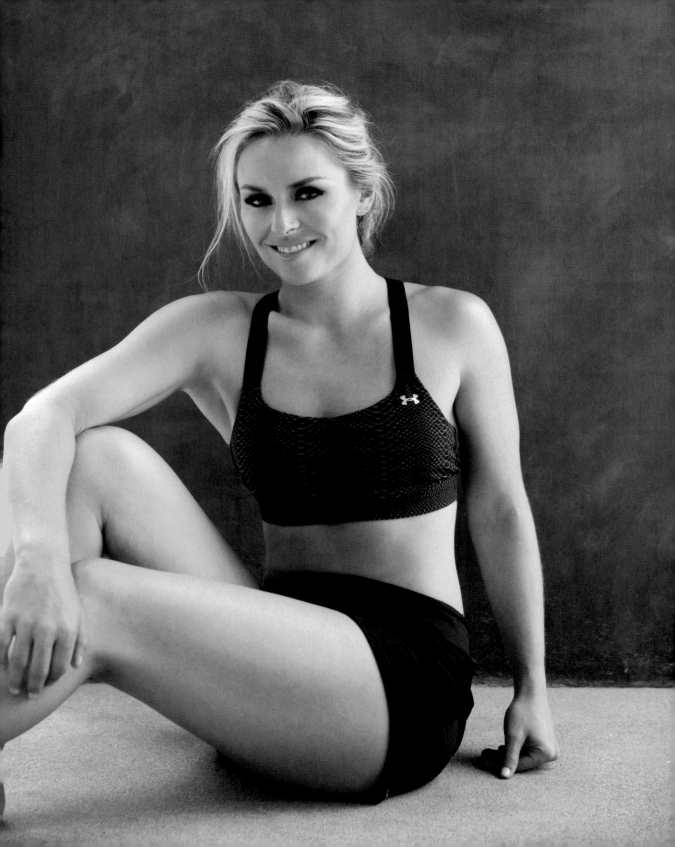

1/
THE POWER
OF STRONG

'm a professional alpine ski racer—I have been since I was fifteen. I love my sport, I love spending time up in the mountains, and I love the feeling of going fast and controlling every muscle in my body to carve around gates while throttling down mountain faces steeper than the stairs in the Empire State Building.

I also love my body—it's what's allowed me to do my sport and to do it well. And I've learned to love the way my body looks, even though my physical appearance has changed during my career as an elite athlete. At times, I've been trim and toned, while on other occasions, I've looked thicker and less muscular. I've gained and lost fat, I've built and rebuilt muscle, I've put on and dropped water weight, and I've injured myself to the point of being unable to move for months, only days after winning races. I've stood on Olympic podiums, walked red carpets, appeared on countless television shows, been on magazine covers, and made the pages of swimsuit issues. I haven't always felt great about how my body looks, but through it all, I've always loved my body.

But today I love how my body looks more than I ever have—and not just because I'm more toned (which I am), but because I've learned how to eat and work out to make my body stronger than it's ever been before, both inside and out.

The reason I wanted to write this book is to share with you my journey to get strong so that I can help you, too, look and feel better than you have ever before, whether you're heavy or skinny, thin-hipped or full-figured, short or tall, or somewhere in between. I believe that every body is beautiful and strong. And if you learn how to leverage that beauty and strength while eating clean and exercising right, you'll look and feel better than you ever have before, whether your goal is to lose weight, boost your health, or simply look fabulous in a bathing suit, a little black dress, or your baggiest pair of pj's.

How exactly can this book help you?

First, this isn't a typical diet book. I don't believe in diets; many will only make you miserable, not thinner and certainly not healthier. I know because I've tried nearly every diet there is—low-carb, high-carb, all-protein, no-sugar, and nearly everything in between. And what I've learned after many trials, tribulations, and times of utmost despondency is that dieting just doesn't work.

Second, this isn't a typical exercise book. I don't believe that there's one way to work out or one type of exercise that will make everyone fabulously skinny, ridiculously toned, and superbly happy. Instead, I believe that there's an exercise or workout program perfect for you that will transform your body—once you find and adopt it. I call this finding your Fitness You, and it's one of the best ways to get strong and lean. I found my Fitness Me through skiing, cycling, and strength training, and it's helped make me stronger and leaner, as well as healthier and happier.

Here's what you'll learn in this book:

- How to eat to get strong and lean and to look better naked without ever counting calories, giving up carbs, never drinking coffee again, or going on some other crazy diet plan

- A one-week step-by-step food plan to help you stop eating processed junk and start eating healthy, fat-burning foods

- My favorite easy-to-make meals and snacks that will help you drop unhealthy weight and add muscle

- A step-by-step plan to find your Fitness You so you can start doing workouts you love to help your body look and feel its best

- How to work out at home in minutes without a DVD, personal trainer, or expensive exercise equipment

- Sixty-five of my favorite Get Strong exercises, with instructional photos and detailed descriptions

- Nine different circuits that you can do anywhere, anytime, no matter your job or daily schedule

Throughout this book, I emphasize getting strong, not getting thin or losing lots of weight. I don't believe women need to be thin to be beautiful—I'm not supermodel thin, after all, and I still think I'm beautiful. What's more, not everyone has the genes or even the ability to lose a ton of weight and whittle down to a size 4—nor should everyone necessarily try for health reasons.

Why make it your goal to get strong and share this amazing adventure with me? There are many reasons to get strong, but here are five major benefits you can see if you commit to transforming your eating and exercise habits with me:

1 **YOUR SELF-CONFIDENCE WILL TRIPLE.** The stronger I am, the more confident I feel—it's that simple. When I exercise and eat right, I'm tighter, sleeker, and sexier, and I feel like all of my muscles are working efficiently and effectively together. I can feel my metabolism firing, and I'm hungry for healthy foods that I know will fuel, not fatten, my body.

When I don't work out or eat right, on the other hand, I feel pretty terrible—physically, mentally, and emotionally. I'm low in energy, I hunch forward, I crave junk, I can lose my motivation to work out, and I don't have that same spark for life that I usually have. Worse, I can start to feel uncomfortable in my own body and question myself, like whether I can really pull off a tight-fitting dress or even keep winning trophies, titles, and medals.

If you're thinking, *She's an Olympic skier. Of course she feels more confident working out and eating right!,* you should know that strength is not a confidence booster for athletes only. I've seen friends, family, even women I don't know at my home gym in Vail become more confident when they eat and work out to get strong rather than to get thin or reach an arbitrary number on the scale. Because getting strong isn't just a physical goal: It's a mental and emotional one, too—an objective that can empower you to get more out of life, whether you want to ski faster like me or simply achieve whatever you set your mind and body to do.

DID YOU KNOW?
What Feels Better Than Losing Weight

Making it your goal to get strong can boost your confidence as much as becoming fit or even losing a ton of weight, according to research. Studies show that people feel significantly better about themselves and how they look simply when they start to work out regularly, regardless of whether they drop a single pound or get any fitter as a result.

2 YOU WILL FEEL MORE BEAUTIFUL AND SEXY, NO MATTER YOUR SIZE OR SHAPE. In my opinion—and in the opinion of most people I know—a strong body is a beautiful body. I love how muscular my legs, butt, arms, and abs look, and how eating clean and working out have helped define my curves. I feel sexier and more feminine when I'm strong, like all my muscles are pulled up together and that my body will look spectacular, regardless of what the bathroom scale says, in any outfit I pull together.

When you commit to getting strong, you agree to go on an incredible journey that will transform your physical appearance as much as it will your physical and mental well-being. Here's how:

- You will add muscle and drop flab without going on a diet or starving yourself.

- You will help your bust look shapelier, your waist trimmer, your thighs leaner, your butt tighter, your arms more sculpted, and your legs longer by adopting a strength-training routine and eating clean.

- You will improve your posture and look taller after just a little time in the weight room.

- You will help your skin look clearer, your hair healthier, and your nails stronger by eating more healthy whole foods.

- You will move more easily and elegantly in everything you do, with better balance and coordination, by eating right and combining some cardio with strength work.

Best of all, when you agree to get strong, you also agree to help your body look as beautiful and sexy as it possibly can in a way that your body will welcome, not fight against.

3 **YOU WILL IMPROVE YOUR HEALTH IN WAYS YOU NEVER KNEW POSSIBLE.** You've heard it before: Eating right and working out are the two best ways to improve your health and protect yourself from low energy, illness, and disease. But not every diet or exercise program will make you healthy. In fact, some diets, as I'll discuss in chapter 2, can actually harm your health, while some workout plans, if they're too intense or poorly structured, won't give you results without boosting your risk of injury and burnout.

Making it your goal to get strong, though, is synonymous with mak-

LINDSEY'S LESSONS

Why You Shouldn't Always Believe What You See

When you flip open a magazine, it's easy to think that everyone has a perfect body—no dimples, sags, cellulite, or other flaws. As a pro athlete, I'm always doing photo shoots for magazines or commercials, and I've learned that there's a big difference between "real" photos and the pictures that end up in magazines and advertisements. Most photos are airbrushed or retouched to remove cellulite and make women look thinner. I was even airbrushed once (and not by choice!) so that my abs looked less muscular. And don't forget about the effect that filters can have on photos you see posted on social media—the right filter used on a photo taken at the right angle can make almost anyone look like a size 2.

ing it your goal to get healthy. When you work to get strong, you eat to give your body all the nutrients it needs for good health, and you don't cut out food groups, starve yourself, eat only processed foods, or adopt other habits that can hurt your health.

When you make it your goal to get strong, you also agree to start exercising in a way that will make your body feel good. You don't go to the gym twice a day, do a bunch of crazy exercises you don't like, or adopt another type of exercise program that will leave you injured, in pain, or unhappy.

Even better, making it your goal to get strong is an intention you can sustain for years, not weeks or months—which is as long as most people can last on restrictive diets or absurd workout plans. And of course, the longer you stay strong, the more you will improve your health.

4 YOU WILL DISCOVER MORE HAPPINESS AND JOY IN YOUR EVERY-
DAY LIFE. Training is hard work. Believe me, there are days when I don't

feel like working out at all and would rather watch *Law & Order* (my favorite TV show) and eat ice cream (my favorite food) on the couch. And while every once in a while I give myself permission to do exactly that, those days are few and far between.

I don't force myself to work out because it's part of my job—I do it because I love it and I know that getting and feeling strong will make me happier. Eating clean and working out have helped me be more optimistic and in the right frame of mind to discover more of the little joys in life—things I don't always see when my mood is clouded by not eating right or exercising.

DID YOU KNOW?

The Natural Way to Boost Your Mood

Studies show that exercise works like an antidepressant, boosting levels of the body's "feel-good" chemical serotonin. In fact, many psychiatrists now prescribe exercise to help treat depression.

Ever heard of runner's high, the euphoria people can feel after working out? (It doesn't happen only after running—I hate running, so I know.) That's what getting strong is like: It makes you high on happiness. In fact, studies show that just one single day of eating healthy and finding some time to exercise can boost your mood significantly.

To get the most joy, though, you should try to find the foods and exercises that will make your individual body feel best. Similar to how not every diet and fitness regimen will make you healthy, not all eating and exercise plans will make you happy. Throughout this book, you'll learn

Getting **Strong** Will Get You **Healthy**

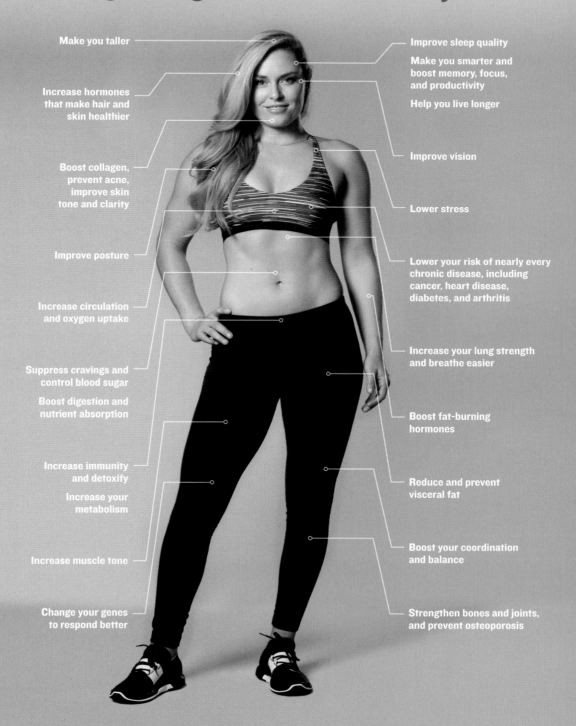

Make you taller

Increase hormones that make hair and skin healthier

Boost collagen, prevent acne, improve skin tone and clarity

Improve posture

Increase circulation and oxygen uptake

Suppress cravings and control blood sugar

Boost digestion and nutrient absorption

Increase immunity and detoxify

Increase your metabolism

Increase muscle tone

Change your genes to respond better

Improve sleep quality

Make you smarter and boost memory, focus, and productivity

Help you live longer

Improve vision

Lower stress

Lower your risk of nearly every chronic disease, including cancer, heart disease, diabetes, and arthritis

Increase your lung strength and breathe easier

Boost fat-burning hormones

Reduce and prevent visceral fat

Boost your coordination and balance

Strengthen bones and joints, and prevent osteoporosis

The Science-Backed Reason It's Good to Break Up with Skinny

Everyone is born with a natural predisposition for a certain type of body. This is why some people are tall and others are short; some are naturally thin while others are bigger boned. Part of this is genetics, of course, but many researchers also believe in something more specific called the set-point theory, the idea that each of us is born with built-in physiological controls dictating how much weight our bodies like to carry. Lose more weight than your set point mandates, and your body will fight it by slowing your metabolism and boosting appetite. Conversely, gain more weight than your set point wants, and your body will try to stymie that weight gain—although most people are immune to this, thanks to the prevalence of supernaturally calorie-dense but nutrient-devoid food in our diets.

The interesting thing about set point, though, is that it shows our bodies function optimally when we're at our natural weight. Maintain your set point, and research shows you'll have more energy, be less likely to get sick, and even feel happier and more optimistic.

If you've tried to get skinny in the past without results, there's a good chance that you physically can't get skinny—your body's set point won't allow it, no matter how little you eat. This is another reason diets can be so ineffective, because your body will plateau at the weight it wants, regardless of how little you eat or how much you exercise.

to tailor my eating and exercise recommendations to suit your likes, dislikes, and lifestyle.

5 **YOU WILL HELP EMPOWER YOUR BODY AND MIND TO SEEK NEW HEIGHTS AND GOALS.** At the very core of this book, I believe that getting strong is all about empowering your body and your mind. When I feel strong, I feel like I can accomplish anything I want. This doesn't mean just winning gold medals or World Cup titles, but also making friends, spending more time with my family, doing all the things I love, and having the confidence and energy to try new things and go on new adventures.

There's something else extremely liberating about getting strong: It has helped me learn to love my body, no matter my size or shape. There are still things I want to improve on physically, mentally, and emotionally, but I'm proud of how I look and of the work that I've put into my body to get it to the point where I can still ski and win races, even after all my crashes and injuries.

———

I can't tell you how to love your body. No one can. Many self-help books make some big guarantees, but in reality, only you know what you need to do to accept and love your body.

What I can do is share my experiences as a woman whose life has been shaped by my body to help show you how to love your own body. This is what getting strong is all about—building strength on the inside as much as on the outside. Because once you learn to love your body, you can do and be anything in the world that you want. I know, because I've done it.

What are you waiting for? Your journey to get strong starts now.

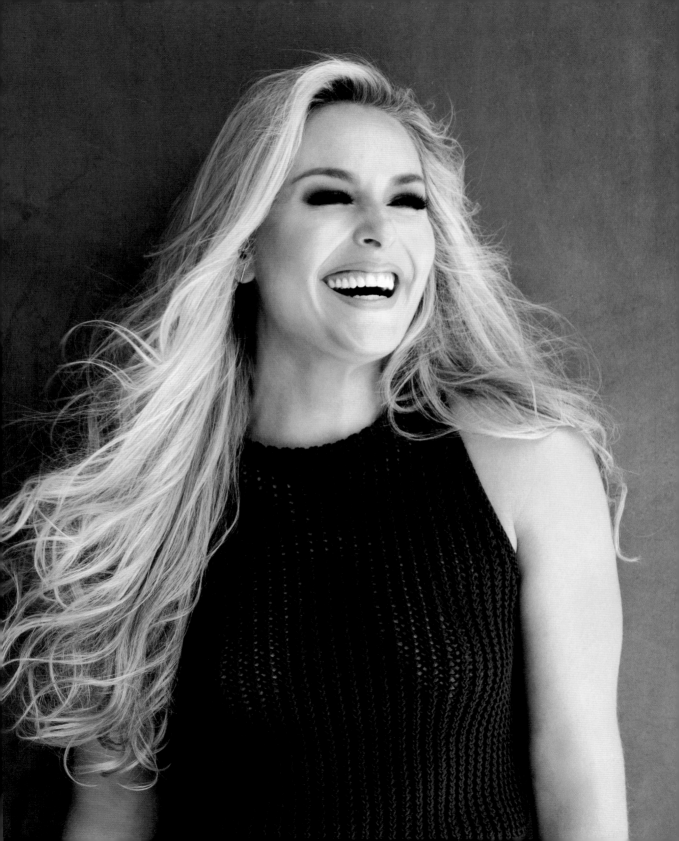

2/ CHANGE YOUR MIND, CHANGE YOUR BODY

Life changes very quickly in a very positive way if you let it.

I once said that to a reporter for *Vogue* magazine, and since then, I've seen it cited as one of my more inspiring maxims. (I was also quoted as saying that I find folding laundry relaxing, but for some curious reason, this hasn't been repeated with the same enthusiasm.)

When it comes to your physical health and appearance, nothing could be more fitting: Your body can and will change quickly in a very positive way if you let it. In short, if you want to change your body, you have to change your mind first, and adopting the right mental attitude is the first step to transforming your body into what you want it to be.

I'd been a strong athlete for years before I really got the body I wanted, and it wasn't until I overhauled how I saw food and my diet that I was able to get as strong and lean as I could.

You may need a new outlook on food, and you may also have to do a mental reset of how you view exercise or your body image—or all three. In my opinion, once you reshape how you see diet, exercise, and physical image, you'll have the mental attitude you need to change your body quickly in a positive way. Here's how.

1 **STOP THINKING YOU HAVE TO GO ON A "DIET" TO LOSE WEIGHT.**
Restrictive diets don't work. I know because I've tried plenty of them in my fifteen-plus years as a professional athlete. Every time, I've had high hopes that cutting carbs, consuming some ridiculous amount of protein, or giving up grains and dairy would help me add muscle, lose fat, and ultimately become a better skier. And nearly every time, I put up with major irritation, inconvenience, hunger, and even some misery only to

discover that I look the same—and feel worse—whenever I control my eating in a restrictive way.

For most people, it's difficult to mentally accept that diets don't work, especially since we've been fed (literally) the opposite by the media and others who make millions selling diet foods and restrictive eating plans. But when you look at the hard facts over time—not just the ephemeral results some celebrities or even a few of your friends may have enjoyed—you'll realize that the majority of people who go on a diet (meaning they adopt an overly restrictive way of eating) can't maintain the weight loss for more than several months. In fact, research shows that 97 percent of all dieters regain any pounds they lose—and then some more—within three years. This startling statistic has led scientists to conclude that one of the biggest predictors of future weight gain is having recently been on a diet. Yikes!

Here are three specific reasons dieting doesn't work:

- **Dieting slows your metabolism.** Going on a restrictive diet or cycling through one diet after another isn't just frustrating—it can also wreak havoc on your metabolism. Studies show that restrictive or yo-yo dieting can slow your resting metabolic rate by as much as 20 percent! This means that if you normally need 1,800 calories per day to maintain your current weight, you would need only 1,440 calories after dieting, thanks to metabolic slowdown. Yet if you go back to eating how much you're used to after being on a diet, you'll put those pounds right back on.

- **Dieting screws up healthy hormone levels.** Restrict how many calories or carbs you eat, and you can interfere with the delicate hormonal balance your body needs to control appetite, burn fat, and build muscle. In particular, dieting causes an uptick in the stress hormone cortisol, which can not only make you feel more tense and irritable but can also boost cravings, hunger, and actual fat storage—a defense mechanism from the days of early humans when stress didn't mean big work deadlines, but going days without food. What's more, elevated cortisol and dieting's other hormonal changes don't necessarily end the day you stop eating a certain way, but can affect your body for up to one year.

- **Most weight loss you see on restrictive diets is water weight.** Most people can lose 5 to 10 percent of their bodyweight in the first few weeks of a restrictive diet. But—and it's a big BUT—almost all that initial weight loss is water, not fat, according to research, which gets released from your cells as your body starts to tap into them for energy. When I tried Paleo, I was excited when I lost some water weight during the first few weeks of the diet, but the results started and stopped there. I didn't lose any fat, and within weeks, that water-weight loss had plateaued.

If you still believe that diets *have* to work—after all, too many experts, magazines, and books tell us they do—so what's the harm in trying, there are actually two big potential harms: Restrictive dieting can jeopardize your physical health and sabotage your mental health. In fact, yo-yo or long-term dieting has been shown to cause low energy, muscle loss, and nutrient deficiencies while increasing your risk of serious conditions such as chronic fatigue, diabetes, heart disease, obesity (as we've seen), and even cancer.

When it comes to your mental health, the research is straightforward: The more you diet, the less likely you are to feel happy. This is not just because dieting in itself is a miserable experience—who likes being hungry all the time? I certainly didn't enjoy it—but because it also lowers levels of the brain's feel-good chemical serotonin.

Dieting's psychological effects don't end at unhappiness, either. Restrictive eating can cause you to develop food addictions, overeating or binge eating, and low self-esteem. The binge-eating part happened to me when I was racing through Italy and was constantly surrounded by delicious-looking bread, pizza, and pasta—all forbidden foods on the Paleo diet. Eventually I couldn't take it anymore, so I told myself that I could have one slice of pizza if I won my next race. Well, I won, and I didn't have just one slice, but an entire large pie. The next morning I woke up feeling gross and nauseous, with an upset stomach that affected my training for several days. I also felt pretty bad about myself—what kind of girl eats an entire large pizza?

Binge eating, along with feelings of guilt and low self-esteem, can have disastrous effects, too. While I eventually snapped out of my pizza-induced reproach, for many chronic dieters, those feelings of guilt and low self-esteem never go away.

2 **IF YOU DON'T BELIEVE EXERCISE CAN BE FUN, YOU HAVEN'T FOUND THE RIGHT WORKOUT FOR YOU.** Plenty of coaches, trainers, and other athletes have told me throughout my career that I should do a certain strength-training move or one kind of cardio workout if I want to be the best possible skier or have the best possible body. And while I'm always eager to try new activities, even those that I don't think I'll like at first, if I'm not enjoying something after several attempts, I don't care how many calories it's burning or what it's doing for my butt or legs—I'm not going to keep doing it unless it's absolutely necessary for my sport. That's be-

DID YOU KNOW?
Dieting Can Make You Look Heavier to Yourself

Dieting for even a few months can lower confidence so much that you can start seeing yourself as heavier than you actually are. Studies show that long-term dieting triggers chemical changes in women's brains that causes them to perceive their bodies as larger than they really are.

The Unbelievable Effects One Diet Had on Thirty-Six Men

One of the most influential studies ever done on dieting was conducted during World War II by a University of Minnesota researcher named Ancel Keys. He put thirty-six healthy men on a 1,600-calorie daily diet, which is pretty typical of most restrictive diets today, in the hopes of having them lose up to 2 pounds per week.

After just a few weeks on the diet, most men reported feeling irritable, dizzy, anxious, and depressed. Over time, they also suffered muscle soreness, hair loss, swelling, and even ringing in their ears. Many became obsessed with food, even though they'd had no previous issues, collecting cookbooks, adding water to meals to make them last longer, and chewing so much gum—up to forty sticks per day—that the researchers eventually had to take it away. One man was pulled from the study after researchers discovered him stealing food scraps from garbage cans, while another became suicidal. Yet another cut off three of his fingers in an act of self-mutilation.

After six months, the men were allowed to return to normal eating, and those feelings of depression and lethargy slowly lifted. But many reported severe hunger, weakness, binge eating, and low libido for months—one man was even hospitalized for bingeing. Moreover, most of the men gained a substantial amount of weight in the year after they stopped the diet, even though they had never been overweight in the past.

cause I've learned that the single most important thing about any exercise program is that you have to love what you do if you want to change your body and maintain those changes over time.

Think it's impossible to love working out? It's not. You just haven't discovered your Fitness You, or the way of working out that makes you immensely happy. In chapter 7, I'll tell you everything you need to know to find your Fitness You, but before you start on your journey, you need to change the way you look at exercise. In short, stop thinking of it as a chore and start viewing at it as something that can give you a good deal of satisfaction—in more ways than one. Because one of the strongest predictors of whether people stick with an exercise program isn't how accommodating their work schedule is, how close the gym is to their home, or how much leisure time they have, but how satisfied they feel about exercise on these following four levels.

- **Yes, working out is fun.** I enjoy the physical sensation of racing down a mountain on skis, my muscles tense but in control. I also like the gritty feeling of lifting weights in the gym—it's that same combination of control and tension. To me, these activities are fun, and I enjoy myself in the moment. And this is the very first condition of any workout: It can and should be fun. Sure, exercise can be challenging, difficult, and even physically uncomfortable at times, but overall, it should give you pleasure. Accept that there is a way of moving your body on a regular basis that will make you happy, and you're halfway to finding your Fitness You.

- **Whatever exercise you do should make you feel strong.** When I walk off the hill or out of the weight room, I feel fitter, stronger, and more muscular—and these are such rewarding feelings that they keep me coming back for more. Whatever workout you choose should make you feel similar. While you shouldn't expect to walk away feeling stronger the first few times you try anything, if an exercise isn't making your body feel physically better over time, keep looking—you can and will find one that does if you let it happen.

- **Your workout should be a mental boost, not a drain.** Skiing and weight lifting tone my mind as much as they do my body, helping me feel calmer, clearer, and sharper. If exercise doesn't give you a similar mental boost right now, don't worry: It can, but you must be willing to search for a way of exercising that will make you feel both mentally strong and physically strong.

- **Your workout can make you feel good about you.** When I'm on the hill or in the weight room, I get this look on my face that says, *Don't mess with* *me*. I know what I'm doing, and I feel capable, competent, and self-assured. This is how your workout can and should make you feel, and it's important to find a form of exercise that does just that. Not only does this give you a great opportunity to feel like a badass on a regular basis, but the more proficient you feel doing an exercise, the more likely you are to stick with it.

Of course, no one tries a new machine, a different lifting move, or an unfamiliar sport and knows exactly what she's doing right away. And you don't have to! That's what's great about new workouts: You get to be a novice and throw your arms and legs around like you have no idea what you're doing—because you don't. But if you want something to stick, at some point, you should feel like you're good at what you're doing. This doesn't mean you need to be the fastest skier on the hill or the most flexible yogi in the class. But you should be open to finding a way of exercising that makes you feel competent, not necessarily superlative.

3 **MENTALLY BREAK UP WITH THE MYTH THAT YOU HAVE TO BE SKINNY TO BE BEAUTIFUL.** Everywhere I look these days—magazines, movies, TV, advertisements for everything from doughnuts to dish soap—it seems that you have to be skinny to be beautiful. In my opinion, though, every body is beautiful—skinny or heavy, curvy or straight, muscular or not. If you really want to help your body get strong on the outside, you first have to make it strong on the inside, which means that you may have to give up the idea that you have to be skinny to be beautiful.

For me, I could never be super skinny and be a professional skier—racers need muscle mass to maneuver around gates and handle the high speeds of the sport. But more important, I would never *want* to be super skinny. I like the way my body looks just the way it is, and I think that I have a beautiful body, muscle mass and all.

I know that you have a beautiful body too, whether you're super skinny, have lots of muscle like me, or are all soft curves and cleavage. It's taken me years to learn and accept this, but I now know that there is no one-size-fits-all when it comes to what's attractive and appealing. Beautiful women are short, tall, big-busted, flat-chested, rail thin, regular thin, full-figured, pear-shaped, apple-shaped, and all the varieties of fruit in between.

What matters more than your shape, dress size, or some number on a scale is how you feel about your body—your most precious possession. Because if you love your body and truly believe that you have a beautiful body no matter what size it is, that inner strength will shine through and make you that much more radiant and beautiful.

Confidence is contagious, and when you perceive your own body as beautiful, others see you as beautiful, too.

———

Learning to accept your body, just the way you are now, isn't easy, but it is the best part about getting strong. No matter how much muscle you add or fat you lose or how totally hot you can look in a little black dress by the end of this book, the most powerful, enduring, and life-shaping strength you can ever build is the one of self-love. Your physical body is fleeting, after all—we all lose muscle, we all grow old, and what we look like now is never what we can look like ten years from now, thanks to age and fate.

Love, on the other hand, is everlasting and can conquer all, as cliché as that may be. And if you can learn to love yourself, you will be beautiful on the inside and out, no matter how you age or your body changes, forever and ever.

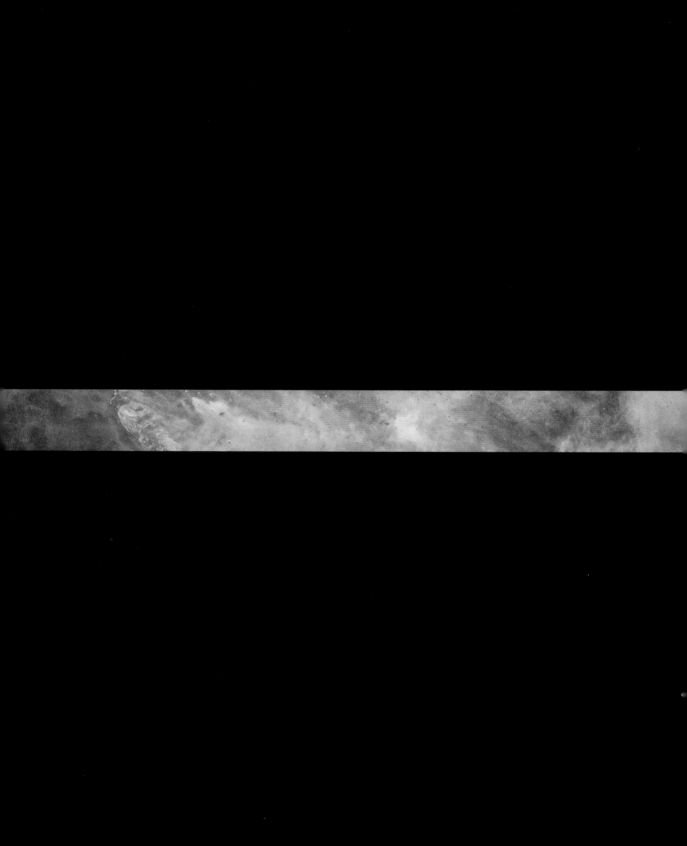

DIET

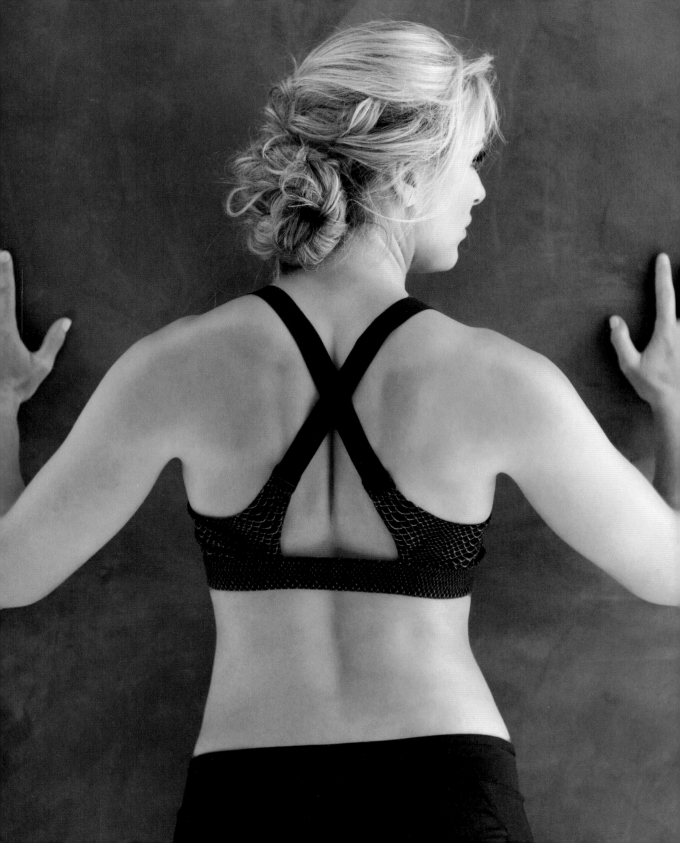

3/ HOW TO EAT TO GET STRONG

A few years after I joined the ski team, I moved to an apartment in Park City with three of my teammates, all guys. You might expect that in a house full of Olympic-level athletes, our kitchen would look like something from the pages of a cookbook on healthy living, but nothing could have been further from the truth. Instead, the guys stocked the kitchen with doughnuts, pasta, pizza, soda, candy, and store-bought cakes. They ate sugary cereal for breakfast, made white-bread sandwiches for lunch, and polished off pints of ice cream at night. Hardly any of us cooked, except to boil water for spaghetti and microwave jarred meat sauce to complete the meal.

We weren't eating this way because we were lazy, trying to be lazy, or simply unschooled in nutritional trends. Quite the opposite; we thought we were following the best diet that we could at the time to build muscle, fortify our bodies for long hours of grueling training, and improve our overall performance as skiers. Carbo-loading was a popular approach for many elite athletes, especially skiers, who require a greater degree of muscle mass to train and race.

But carbo-loading never made me feel strong, and it certainly didn't make me add muscle or lose the fat I wanted. Instead, I felt weak and tired, my face grew puffier and puffier, and whenever I caught a glimpse of myself in the mirror, I thought that I looked less toned, even though I was working out for hours every day.

It took me years to figure out a way to eat that would help me look and feel good. As an elite athlete, I'm always looking for the best new way to get that extra edge—the one little push that will help lift me from world-class athlete to top of the world. So for the past fifteen years, I've tried different diets, trends, and fads in the effort to make my body as strong and lean as physically possible. A handful have offered some benefits, but none made the significant, sustainable changes to my body that I hope for—until I found the one approach that has nothing to do with dieting or fads and everything to do with science and the foods that have helped people get strong and lean for centuries.

———

When I was growing up in Minnesota, my parents both worked full time, and like most families in Middle America, we ended up eating a lot of processed foods: sugary cereal, ready-to-eat dinners, Hamburger Helper, and grilled cheeses with canned soup, supplemented by a few great meals my father would make on the weekends. But we rarely ate any veggies, and when we had to, I secretly slipped them under the table to our dog, Thunder. When I went away to ski camps, I'd often just have a pint of ice cream and call it a meal.

I didn't give too much thought to what I ate when I was young, especially since my habit of eating ice cream for dinner didn't seem to be impeding my career as a junior skier. But after the 2002 Olympics, when I was seventeen, I suddenly gained twenty-five pounds in one summer. My metabolism had changed, even though I was still training several hours each day. I was both surprised and disheartened, but it was one of the first of what would be many valuable lessons I had to learn on how to get strong: All the exercise in the world can't derail the effects of unhealthy eating.

Shortly after the Olympics, while living with my pasta-loving teammates in Park City, I began a high-carb diet, eating foods like bagels and pancakes for breakfast, starchy energy bars and sandwiches for lunch, and, on some nights, an entire box of spaghetti for dinner.

It wasn't until I was in my twenties and started going to summer camps at the Olympic Training Center (OTC) in Chula Vista that I slowly began to discover the power of unprocessed foods. The summer camps attracted Olympic-caliber athletes from all across the country in a range of different disciplines—not just winter sports, but track and field, rowing, soccer, and triathlon. When I walked into the cafeteria for lunch the first day, I realized that I had a rare and amazing opportunity to actually see firsthand what some of the strongest, leanest, and fittest people in the country ate on a regular basis.

So I watched as if I were a researcher in an observational study—and I learned. Many triathletes and track-and-field runners weren't lining up with me for pancakes or pasta, but were ordering eggs or oatmeal in the morning, making their own salads at lunch, and going for grilled meat and vegetables at night.

Seeing how these athletes ate and listening to them talk about how food made them feel—light, energized, and aerodynamic—I resolved to start experimenting. I began by eating eggs and oatmeal for breakfast—two dishes not part of my regular routine—and swapping out some pasta and pizza for chicken and steak. I also started trying to eat more vegetables, which I had previously consumed only when asked (and usually then only if they were doused in butter or garlic). Without Thunder under the table, I was surprised to learn that I actually liked the taste of some.

Almost immediately, I began to see what my runner and triathlete friends had been talking about: I felt lighter, peppier, more focused—as if I could go longer and harder in workouts. The puffiness in my face began to ease, my clothes started to fit a bit better, and I thought that I might be looking more toned when I watched myself doing squats and lunges in the gym mirror.

When I left the training camp, I tried to continue the healthy habits I had learned, but it was difficult. My experiences at the OTC hadn't been long or frequent enough to impart lasting changes, and as I started to travel more to race and train, it was easy to fall back into old habits, especially since many sports nutritionists still recommended lots of pasta and other heavy carbs.

At the same time, more of my teammates were moving away from the high-carb approach to consuming more protein and began supplementing with daily protein shakes. I started drinking them too, because I also wanted more protein, and the shakes seemed to be a good way to ensure a steady supply without relying on the creamy chicken or butter-glazed seafood dishes that were popular at most European restaurants where we traveled. And while the shakes seemed to help me build muscle, I didn't exactly feel clean, light, and energized when chugging back a concentrated dose of processed protein powder.

At one point in my twenties, as I continued to struggle to find a way to eat that would help me get strong no matter what was going on in my life, I convinced myself that if I controlled my diet down to every last bite, I would finally lose the puffiness in my face, become as toned as I had ever hoped, and ski amazingly. So I bought a food scale and began weighing all my meals and snacks and eating every two hours on the hour. As you can imagine, this was time-consuming and entirely unpleasant, and after several months of the routine, I stopped when I realized that not even this degree of dietary regulation was improving my body or my performance.

Then, something happened that altered my mind-set—and consequently my diet—for months: I won a gold medal at the 2010 Olympics. Suddenly I found myself in the spotlight of the American media. I was invited to Hollywood parties, got asked to attend celebrity events, and was doing back-to-back TV appearances and magazine features.

Going to premieres and walking the red carpet both thrilled and terrified me. I loved getting dressed up and meeting new people, but at the same time, I felt taller, bigger, and more muscular than the other women there. For the first time in my career, I began to wonder if I needed to be thinner to be successful as an athlete, if that was what was necessary to stay socially and culturally relevant as a woman. I began to view my body and my diet differently, and I grew more concerned with how what I ate would affect my physical appearance than my performance.

At the same time, the Paleo diet—consuming only meat, vegetables, nuts, and some fruit, with no grains, beans, starches, or dairy—was starting to gain traction among some elite athletes, especially my track-and-field friends. When they told me that they felt leaner and faster on the diet than ever before, I was immediately intrigued and decided to try it.

A few weeks after I started the diet, I thought that I'd finally hit the bonanza of nutritional approaches. For the first time since I was seventeen, I lost the puffiness from my face, and I felt quicker and leaner, stronger in the gym, and more confident on the red carpet and in front of a camera. For the first time in my life, I was also consuming nearly no processed foods—no shakes, bars, microwave meals, sugary stuff, or refined grains—and that influx of clean, healthy whole foods was working wonders on my body and mind.

But the good feelings didn't last long. Because I wasn't eating starchy carbs, my energy began to flag and my workouts started to suffer. The plan was difficult to sustain, whether I was on the road or at home, and I started eating the same thing every day only because I felt like I didn't have many other options: hard-boiled eggs and raw red bell peppers for breakfast, and grilled, baked, or roasted meat with a side of steamed vegetables for lunch *and* for dinner. Nothing tasted good to me, and I began to lose interest in eating, even though I was hungry most of the time. I started to crave foods that I hadn't longed for in years while missing healthy items like yogurt, oatmeal, and potatoes that weren't allowed on the diet.

Eventually, after months of eating strict Paleo, I started to have intense cravings for carbs—not just the occasional hankering here and there, but a continual yearning for pasta, pizza, bread, and other decidedly non-Paleo foods that I saw everywhere I went through Europe on the World Cup circuit.

Then, in the winter of 2011, after nearly two years on the diet and in the middle of consecutive World Cup races, I couldn't take it anymore. I was tired, miserable, and hungry, and I couldn't stomach the idea of another hard-boiled egg (I was eating up to eight at a time). I went down to the hotel restaurant and ordered muesli—and with the first bite, I felt like I was eating delicious bliss in a bowl. Later that day, whether psychosomatic or not, I felt fueled up to attack my workout and thought that my body finally had the nutrients it needed to be strong.

That one bowl of muesli broke my nearly two-year streak on the Paleo diet. Immediately after, I began eating more oats and bread and experimenting with adding carbs like quinoa and wild rice that had never been part of my diet before. At the same time, I knew that I felt stronger eating mostly whole foods thanks to my tenure on Paleo, and I made a big effort to pick out only whole-grain bread and other items—not the enriched wheat flour bread, flavored oatmeal, and white rice and pasta that take up most of the space on supermarket shelves. I also began to prioritize a macronutrient that had never been the central focus of my diet: fat. I stocked up on avocados, nuts, different types of

DID YOU KNOW?
You May Be Eating More Chemicals Than You Think

The average person is exposed to approximately 10 to 13 pesticides a day through food and drink, 90 percent of which have been linked to weight gain.

olive oil, and full-fat dairy, and tried eating more fat during the day while supplementing with carbs on other occasions.

Over the next several years, through a series of additions, assessments, subtractions, and tweaks, I finally hit upon a food plan that worked. It was helping me get stronger, leaner, and incredibly toned. What I was doing was simple—just eating whole foods with a balance of carbs, protein, and fat—but it was giving my body everything it needed and none of the processed junk that it didn't. I wasn't counting calories, cutting out food groups, suffering ridiculous cravings, eating mostly one type of macronutrient, or going hungry. This wasn't a regimented diet, and as I discovered with time, whole foods can be found abundant everywhere when you know where to look, so I could eat this way anywhere at any time, whether traveling through Europe, training at home, or dining out with friends or family. Today this is how I eat: clean, healthy, balanced, and whole. This one easy, simple strategy has transformed my body in some ways I always wanted and in others I never expected.

If you're ready to start eating to feel better, look better, and become stronger, leaner, and more toned than you ever have been before, come along with me, and I'll show you how clean eating can transform your body and life, too.

The Scientific Proof for Unprocessed Foods

As you can imagine, tons of research has been conducted on what causes people to gain and lose weight—after all, weight loss is a $40 billion annual industry. That said, you can find at least one study showing some benefit to almost any diet—high-carb, low-carb, vegan, raw, all-cookie, or even a bacon-and-steak-only approach.

The truth is, there is *some* short-term benefit to almost every diet (with the exception maybe of the all-cookie diet). But when you look at

Eat Like Lindsey: A Day of Clean Eating

Breakfast: Eggs scrambled with salsa, avocado, onions, and mushrooms; steel-cut oatmeal

Snack: Full-fat Greek yogurt with chopped nuts

Lunch: Spinach salad with roasted chicken, quinoa, avocado, and mixed nuts

Snack: Whole-grain English muffin with nut butter and sliced banana

Dinner: Salmon pan-cooked in garlic and olive oil with asparagus

what *really* works, what's healthy, and what's sustainable over a period of time (and ignore studies funded by food companies or conducted on only a handful of people), you'll find one overarching commonality: Prioritizing fresh, whole, unprocessed food, no matter the source or macronutrient makeup, is the best way to lose weight, build muscle, and optimize your physical and mental health.

It may sound simple, and really it is, but whole foods are something few people eat today. Instead, the average American gets a whopping 70 percent of her daily calories from processed foods like refined bread, pasta, cereal, chips, candy, and other snacks. Compare that to a hundred years ago, when people consumed almost no processed foods (because they didn't exist) and were much leaner as a result.

What's wrong with processed foods? Food manufacturers process foods to make them last longer on store shelves, be easier or faster to consume without any preparation, and/or have certain flavor combinations, colors, or textures not found in fresh food. When companies process a food, they strip its natural nutrients and add one or more of the following ingredients or chemicals: sugar or other synthetic sweeteners like high-fructose corn syrup; refined grains like enriched wheat flour; hydrogenated oil or other man-made fats; preservatives; artificial colors and flavors; emulsifiers; artificial sweeteners; and so on and so forth. The list goes on. Most of these ingredients and chemicals have no nutritional value, yet are high in calories. What's more, many have been shown to spike blood sugar and disrupt healthy hormone levels, both of which can lead to weight gain. Here are some of the best reasons for choosing whole foods over processed.

- **Whole foods have more nutrition than processed food.** Every single whole food—anything grown out of the earth or raised on a farm that's had little done or added to it before it lands on a store shelf or in your mouth—is high in either fiber, protein, or fat, and contains some naturally occurring vitamins, minerals, and/or antioxidants.

  While some processed foods can be fortified to contain more protein, fiber, vitamins, probiotics, omega-3s, and whatever other nutrients are trending at the time, our bodies don't absorb fortified nutrition as well as what's naturally found in whole foods. This means that when you eat whole foods, you get more nutrients that are bioavailable, meaning your body can use and absorb them.

  Why is good nutrition important? While the answer should be obvious—unhealthy diet and inactivity are the leading causes of death in the United States, according to the government—many people desperate to lose weight seem to unknowingly overlook the importance of good nutrition, thinking that nutrient-poor processed foods like low-cal frozen meals, snacks, and other "diet" foods will help them drop fat. Nothing could be more inaccurate: Without bioavailable nutrition from whole foods, your body can't regulate appetite, build muscle tone, or burn fat as effectively.

- **Quality—not the number of calories, carbs, or grams of protein—is the most important factor in food.** What matters more than the calories, carbs, protein, or fat your diet contains is the quality of those calories if you want to lose weight, according to major obesity studies. If you eat mostly processed foods, research shows that you'll have a harder time feeling full, controlling cravings, building muscle, and losing fat, mostly because you're not getting the good nutrition you need from the calories you're eating.

Why Sugar Is So Bad for You—and the One Easy Way to Cut Back

Perhaps the biggest reason processed foods are so harmful to your health and waistline is that up to three-quarters of them contain added sugar or sweeteners to boost flavor. What's so awful about added sugar? Sure, it's high in calories, but that's not necessarily why sugar is detrimental—after all, lots of healthy whole foods like nuts, avocados, and olive oil are also energy dense.

Instead, when you eat foods that contain added sugar and/or refined grains (which are made up of sugar), that sugar enters your bloodstream quickly, triggering the body to release the hormone insulin. Insulin helps sop up sugar in the blood by storing what it can't use immediately for energy as fat in your cells. As if that weren't bad enough, when all that sugar leaves your bloodstream, you can start to feel tired, lethargic, and hungry again, even if you just ate. Added sugar has also been shown to create triglycerides (unhealthy blood fats), raise "bad" LDL cholesterol, boost blood pressure, and even help accelerate the growth of cells, including potential cancer cells.

For these reasons, a growing number of studies shows that added sugar can increase the risk of nearly every health condition, from premature aging, low libido, depression, and weight gain to more serious problems such as chronic inflammation, diabetes, arthritis, obesity, heart disease, and even cancer.

While I don't believe that you have to cut sugar completely from your diet—doing so can set you up for cravings and binge eating—it's one of the strongest reasons to curb your consumption of processed foods: Research shows that simply swapping whole for processed foods in your diet cuts your sugar intake enough to cause weight loss, even if that's not your goal.

On the other hand, if you eat a diet of mostly clean foods with few processed items, regardless of how many calories or carbs you consume, you'll help stabilize your blood sugar levels, curb cravings, prevent overeating, boost your metabolism, increase your energy, improve your sleep quality, build muscle, and ramp up your body's fat-burning ability.

- **Eating fresh, whole foods burns more calories.** By definition, processed foods contain ingredients that have been refined, or broken down from their natural state. This means that your body digests these foods more quickly. But this quicker breakdown isn't a good thing. Processed foods require less energy (read: calories) to break down. They enter your bloodstream more quickly, causing your blood sugar to spike. This triggers a commensurate response in the hormone insulin, which can stimulate your cells to store that sugar as fat while increasing your feelings of hunger, even if you just ate. Finally, processed foods leave your stomach more quickly, taking any sensation of satisfaction that you had from eating your processed fare with them.

  The energy you burn by choosing whole foods over processed ones is not insignificant by any means. Studies show that whole foods require up to 50 percent more calories to digest than refined junk. This, in theory, can turn a 100-calorie apple into a 50-calorie one, while a 100-calorie bag of cookies will still be 100 calories—and will do more to promote weight loss when you consider the fattening effects that refined flour and sugar can have on your body.

- **Processed foods can cause the same type of addiction as drugs and alcohol.** Can't stop eating after one handful of chips? You're not alone—but don't blame it on your lack of willpower. According to research, potato chips, pizza, chocolate, cookies, and ice cream are the top five most addictive foods and have been shown to be just as habit-forming as hard drugs and alcohol.

  How could this be? These foods, along with the other processed ones that top the ten-most-addictive list, contain concentrated amounts of both fat and sugar—either in the form of actual sugar or the sugar that makes up the building blocks of refined carbs like white flour.

  This concentrated fat-sugar cocktail is artificial, created by food manufacturers to boost taste and texture. For proof, try to think of any one whole food that naturally contains high amounts of sugar and fat. Not only is the combination man-made, it's also harmful, triggering the same type of cravings and withdrawal symptoms that drugs and alcohol cause. This addiction can manifest as overeating, binge eating, weight gain, and obesity, all of which have increased in incidence since the onset of processed foods.

• **Processed foods contain chemicals that can cause weight gain.** Refined products often contain ingredients treated with pesticides, insecticides, animal antibiotics and hormones, and other toxins. Not only are these chemicals bad for the environment, they're also bad for your health, with the ability to slow metabolism and disrupt hormone balance.

In short, eating processed foods often means consuming chemicals that not only interfere with your overall health, but can also thwart your efforts to eat to get strong and lean.

———

There are other reasons it's important to avoid refined foods and eat those closer to the earth, including that it's better for your overall health, better for the environment, and in general, better for local economies when you choose fresh food that can't be sourced from faraway places.

But knowing all the reasons why natural foods are optimal doesn't make cutting out the processed stuff a snap—after all, most of us are addicted to some sugary or refined foods. Still, it doesn't have to be so difficult to swap out processed fare for more healthy, fat-burning foods when you have a game plan, which is exactly what you'll find in the next chapter: my simple five-step strategy to start eating less processed foods and to focus more on the foods your body wants, needs, and will learn to crave to get strong and lean.

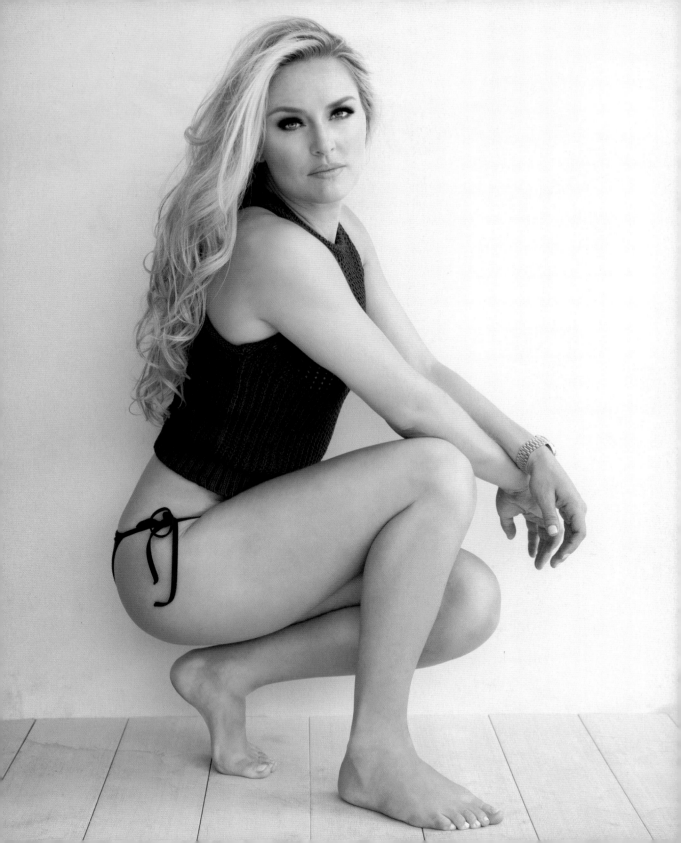

4/
FIVE STEPS TO START EATING LEAN

For much of my twenties, I worked and traveled with a trainer who told me I shouldn't eat chocolate. I loved chocolate—I still do—and while I tried to follow his advice, there were definitely days when I felt like I needed a few squares of good chocolate to make it through a hectic day of traveling, training, or racing schedule. But whenever I admitted to wanting some, he would make me feel guilty, like there was something wrong with me for craving a little chocolate.

Over time, as my guilt increased, so did my cravings, to the point where I started secretly buying chocolate at gas stations and eating entire bars in their bathrooms. Disgusting, right? But, as I now know, obsessive cravings, binge eating, and other unhealthy habits around food can develop when you make certain foods off-limits and don't have a smart plan to deal with the addictive foods that make up the majority of our diets.

What else I've learned in my years as an elite athlete: Chocolate can absolutely be part of any healthy diet when you stop eating junk and start giving your body the whole-foods nourishment it needs. When you add more natural, healthy foods and subtract the sugar and processed stuff from your diet—without denying yourself the things you love that make eating enjoyable—you end up with a satisfying formula for fewer cravings, less guilt, less overeating, and zero weight gain that equals a delicious, fat-burning, muscle-building way to eat.

In this chapter, I've detailed my five-step plan to help you give up a traditional diet of refined foods for one of balanced, healthy nourishment that will still allow you to eat what you love and get strong and lean.

———

You would think that following a diet of only whole foods would be ridiculously easy. And maybe it would be—if we all lived a hundred years ago or in the remote mountain towns I pass through when I'm racing in Europe, where there are few supermarkets, gas stations, fast-food places, or chain restaurants (and consequently, few overweight people).

But for most of the Western world, processed, refined, and fast foods are everywhere, while fresh or whole foods are increasingly difficult to find. More than 60 percent of foods sold on supermarket shelves today are highly processed and contain more fat, sugar, and salt than recommended by international health organizations. What's more, most restaurant and takeout meals are made up of mostly processed ingredients. Combine these facts and you can see why, as I mentioned earlier, processed foods make up an astounding 70 percent of the average American's diet. So for most people, including healthy athletes, it's extremely challenging to eat mostly whole foods.

After ten years of trying, I've learned how to break through that everyday routine and the social norm to eat more whole foods, but it's taken lots of trial and error. Along the way, I've discovered five crucial steps that will make whole-foods eating a whole lot easier for you.

Start by learning these five steps on how to eat clean. Then take my one-week Eat to Get Strong challenge in chapter 5. At the end of one week, eating healthy whole foods will be easy and enjoyable—and you'll be stronger, leaner, healthier, and happier to boot.

1 LEARN THE DIFFERENCE BETWEEN "HEALTHY" AND CLEAN. You can't eat clean if you don't know what it is—or more accurately, what it's not. This may sound obvious, but I used to think that many "healthy" foods were clean only to discover that they contained funky ingredients, were overly processed, or were loaded with added sugar.

Consider yogurt, for example. Nutritionists tout yogurt as a healthy high-protein food that can help you build strong bones, boost digestion, and lose weight. All this is true when you eat plain unsweetened yogurt. But pick yogurt high in added sugar, preservatives, or artificial sweeteners, flavors, and/or colors—most kinds of yogurt on the store shelves today—and it won't help you get strong and lean. If anything, processed yogurt can spike blood sugar, increase hunger, trigger cravings, and interfere with hormone balance, thanks to added sugars and/or artificial ingredients.

Here's another example: bread, probably the food dieters see as the worst. True, most bread items in stores today are high in sugar since they're made from refined or enriched flours and contain added sugar, synthetic emulsifiers, and artificial preservatives. Because refined or enriched flours come from grains stripped of their nutrient-rich bran and germ, processed bread products are also low in fiber, protein, vitamins, and minerals.

Whole-grain bread, on the other hand, is made from the entire grain—bran and germ included—and is high in fiber, protein, and other stomach-filling, fat-burning nutrients. Breads made with whole grains don't boost blood sugar or stimulate cravings like refined-grain breads do, and they can be part of any diet to get strong and lean when you know how to choose the healthiest among them.

Yet figuring out the best type of bread and other healthy whole foods to buy takes work—unless, of course, you're picking up only fresh and unpackaged items, such as raw vegetables, raw meat, whole seafood, and fresh eggs. Otherwise, you have to read a product's ingredients list to make sure that whatever you're getting off the shelves is made up of only whole-food ingredients, without a staggering amount of sugar, refined flour, hydrogenated fat, and other additives shown to cause weight gain.

Thankfully, reading an ingredients list takes only ten seconds once you know how. Write down the following five steps, put them in your phone, or do whatever you have to, because once you can learn to assess whether items are made with whole foods, any grocery store becomes a cornucopia of whole-food goodies that are just as tasty and convenient as the processed stuff.

1. **Assess for length.** If an ingredients list looks longer than you would expect—fifteen items in a box of oatmeal, say—go with your gut and put it back on the shelf. In general, the fewer ingredients a food has, the closer it is to its natural state.

2. **Skim for weird words.** Notice any long, polysyllabic ingredients that you couldn't picture in nature—things like butylated hydroxyanisole, acesulfame potassium, soy lecithin, polysorbates, or high-fructose corn syrup? Reshelve it. But if you can imagine all the ingredients in a product as whole foods sitting on your kitchen counter or growing in a field somewhere, continue to step 3.

3. **Scan for added sugar.** Sugar is the single most important ingredient to limit in your diet if you want to get strong—read why on page 61. Unfortunately, though, cutting back on sugar isn't easy, since it's found in approximately 75 percent of all packaged foods, even those not meant to be sweet. No matter what you buy, check the ingredient list to make sure it doesn't include added sugar. There are sixty different names for the sweet stuff, so it pays to learn the most common aliases for sugar, listed on page 71.

4. **Double-check the sugar grams.** Even though a food might appear to have no added sweeteners, it can still be too high in sugar, thanks to food-based sweeteners such as dried fruit. How many grams per serving are

too many? The World Health Organization recommends consuming no more than 25 grams total per day—only 5 grams more than what's found in one cup of raisin bran cereal. As a general rule, avoid any food that contains more than 15 grams of sugar per serving (unless you're indulging in the occasional treat).

5. **Glance for whole grains.** If you're buying products made from grains like bread, cereal, pasta, or rice, make sure they are made from 100 percent whole grains. What this means is that every flour or grain listed on the ingredient list should be preceded by the word "whole." See the lists opposite to learn how to spot whole grains from refined ones.

2 **STOP TRYING TO FOLLOW A MEAL PLAN—AND START LISTENING TO YOUR BODY.** People are always asking me how much I eat or how much they should eat if they want to get toned and lean. Do you eat two or three eggs in the morning? How much avocado should I add to my salads? Is a cup of rice too much for dinner?

Many weight-loss plans dictate how much you should eat, right down to the quarter cup of romaine to add to your salad or the specific number of nuts to enjoy as an afternoon snack. And while it helps to become more aware of appropriate portion sizes, controlling your food down to the quarter cup and individual nut doesn't encourage a healthy relationship with food. In fact, restrictive or measured meal plans prevent you from listening to your body and learning how to eat intuitively.

In my early twenties, I weighed all my food and ate only exact portion sizes every two hours. When I now look back on this behavior, I realize that it was neurotic, and at the time, it made me miserable. And despite all the effort, the plan did nothing to change my body. Then, when I stopped the plan, I had a difficult time discerning when I was actually hungry and when I was full—two natural instincts that restrictive diets can all but eradicate.

Identify Whole Grains

Don't be fooled by marketing claims on grain-based products that say things like "made with whole grains," "100% wheat," "12 grain," or "multigrain." These claims don't actually guarantee that a product is made with 100 percent whole grains. Instead, read the ingredients list, and look only for names listed below that are whole grains. If a product contains a refined grain on the second list, even if the first ingredient is a whole grain, find one that is made from 100 percent whole grains.

WHOLE GRAINS

Brown rice	Stone-ground whole wheat	Whole-grain triticale
Buckwheat	Wheat berries	Whole oat flour
Bulgur	Whole brown rice flour	Whole quinoa
Cracked whole wheat	Whole-grain barley	Whole rye
Millet	Whole-grain corn	Whole wheat
Oats, oatmeal (including instant and rolled)	Whole-grain sorghum	Wild rice

REFINED GRAINS

All-purpose flour	Degerminated flour	Wheat flour
Bran	Enriched wheat flour	Wheat germ
Cornmeal or corn flour	Malted barley flour	White rice
Cracked wheat	Stone-ground wheat flour	Unbleached flour

Spot Secret Sugars

Added sugar can be found in packaged food under more than sixty different names. Here are twenty-six common aliases that you should know and avoid:

Brown rice syrup	Evaporated cane juice	Panela
Cane juice	Fruit juice concentrate	Panocha
Corn sweetener	Galactose	Raw sugar
Corn syrup	Glucose	Rice (bran) syrup
Crystalline fructose	High-fructose corn syrup	Sorghum
Dextran	Malt syrup	Sucrose
Dextrose	Maltodextrin	Tapioca syrup
Diastatic malt powder	Maltose	Treacle
Ethyl maltol	Oat syrup	

For these reasons, I'm not going to tell you how much you should eat. Instead, I believe you should hone your natural instincts that can tell you when you're hungry and when you're full. That way, you can learn to eat intuitively, listening to your body to discern how much food you need at any given time, in any given situation. When you establish (or reestablish) this critical ability, you take back control of your food and your body. You become less likely to overeat, binge eat, and gain weight. You learn how to consume the right foods in the correct amounts for life, not just because you're forced to as part of a meal plan or restrictive diet. The best part: When you truly embrace intuitive eating, you never gain more weight than your body needs because you will eat only how much your body needs.

Intuitive eating may sound simple—eat when you're hungry, stop when you're full—but it takes a conscientious effort. While we're all born with the physiological cues that tell us when we're hungry and when we're full, most of us lose the ability to hear these cues as we absorb society's culture of food morals, emotions, and rules. We start to eat certain foods and avoid others because we're told that they're good or bad. We consume meals and snacks because we feel lonely, empty, stressed, angry, or bored. Or we eat simply because we are addicted to certain processed foods and crave them.

To relearn to eat when you're hungry, start by asking yourself before every meal and snack whether you're truly hungry—or if you're eating only because it's mealtime, something recently upset you, you're bored or lonely, or you're merely craving a certain food (see page 86 on how to tell hunger from craving). Checking in with your gut—rather than allowing your emotions, cravings, and clock to drive your food consumption—is the first crucial step in intuitive eating.

If your gut tells you that you're still hungry, ask yourself if you've had enough to drink. Many times when I'm hungry, I'm actually dehydrated, which can significantly boost appetite. So I'll have a big glass of water and wait twenty minutes and not feel hungry anymore.

Other times when I think I'm starving, I know that I'm really not. Instead, I only feel that way because I ate something super sugary earlier in the day (or even the night before). Remember, sugar-rich foods can cause a spike in blood sugar and a subsequent surge in insulin that can drive up appetite and hunger for hours. (See the box "Why Sugar Is So Bad for You" on page 61 for more details.) Whenever I realize that I'm suffering from this kind of "fake hunger" after a sugar crash, I'll ignore it or I'll eat something small with protein or fat to help right that sugar-insulin cycle.

The art of discerning when you're full after eating can be more difficult to master. But one of the big benefits of eating mostly whole foods is that you start feeling more full and satisfied from less food because you're giving your body the nutrients it needs to function while consuming more stomach-filling fiber and protein. What's more, when you give up processed sugary junk, you also say good-bye to all those hunger-boosting, appetite-driving additives in food that make us want to eat more and more, no matter how full we might feel. After I started eating a mostly whole-foods diet, I found it became almost second nature to know when I'm full. Today, whenever I'm in doubt, I also use the twenty-minute rule: Wait at least that long after finishing a meal before consuming anything else to give my body time to digest and process. Finally, I always aim to feel full, never stuffed.

3 HEALTHY EATING IS LIKE A HIGH-SCHOOL SCIENCE CLASS: YOU HAVE TO EXPERIMENT. If I had never experimented with my diet, I might still be eating Lucky Charms for breakfast and Hamburger Helper for dinner. My body looks the way it does today because I've learned not only to try new foods but also to experiment with what time of day, how much, and in what combination I eat.

I now eat an avocado every morning, for example, after a nutritionist recommended I add it to my eggs. Since then, I've discovered that the extra fat helps me wake up and focus better. A friend once made me eggs with fresh octopus—a combination some might find odd, if not disgusting—and I was surprised that I liked it. I would probably still be putting octopus in my eggs if it were a more practical everyday ingredient in Colorado.

Because our bodies are all different, some people need to eat more dietary fat to burn fat while others require more carbs or protein to get lean. Experimenting with new dishes and food combinations exposes

TEN SECONDS TO A STRONGER YOU
The Four-Step Checklist Before Eating Anything

1. Do a quick gut check: Is your stomach really empty or are you looking to feed an emotion? Are you upset, bored, or lonely? Or are you eating only because it's mealtime, others around you are, or you saw or smelled something delicious?

2. Use the box about how to tell hunger from craving (see page 86) to discern whether you're really hungry or just suffering a craving.

3. Think back to the last thing you ate. Was it super sugary or high in refined carbs? If so, this could be making you "fake" hungry. Wait it out.

4. Consider what you've had to drink recently. Are you hydrated? If in doubt, try consuming a tall glass of water or other unsweetened beverage and wait twenty minutes before redoing the checklist.

you to varying ratios of macronutrients (protein, fat, and carbs) so that you can find the right proportions for you. By experimenting, I've learned that if I eat more carbs in the morning, I'm never hungry before lunch. But if I eat too many carbs and not enough protein during the day, I start to feel tired and my motivation to work out flags. And since I started eating more fat throughout the day at all my meals, it's been much easier for me to stay leaner and toned.

4 **MAKING CERTAIN FOODS OFF-LIMITS WILL PREVENT YOU FROM GETTING STRONG AND LEAN.** At the beginning of this chapter, I told you about a trainer who said that chocolate was a forbidden food—never to be consumed ever—which only resulted in my craving it more and even binge eating it in bathrooms. After I stopped working with him and chocolate was no longer off-limits, I was surprised to discover that I no longer craved it like I had and that I could eat it like a normal person again, meaning in moderation. Today I'll have a few squares now and then and happily wrap up the rest—no eating (or forcing myself not to overeat) the entire bar. Chocolate isn't a trigger food anymore, but an occasional enjoyable and healthy part of my diet, largely because it's no longer taboo.

It's normal to ascribe moral judgment to foods: *Kale is good, cake is bad. I'm a better person when I eat spinach salads, but I've done something wrong when I eat french fries.* And while moralizing foods can help some people initially make smarter dietary choices, the practice over time usually derails the most disciplined eaters. That's because when you label foods as bad or off-limits, as my trainer did with chocolate, you anoint those foods with a great deal of power. They suddenly become more desirable, more so than when they were "okay" to eat, and you start to crave them, even obsessing over when you can't have them.

When you do indulge in off-limits food, you're more likely to overeat or binge eat, making up for those long-lasting feelings of deprivation. Consequently, you can feel guilty or bad about yourself not just for giving in but also for overeating. This makes it much more likely that you'll decide to just "throw in the towel" on healthy eating for the rest of the day (or even week). You think, *I just ate three chocolate bars in a gas station bathroom, so why not have cake too, and maybe a few bowls of cereal after that?*

For all these reasons, I never tell myself today that I can't eat a certain food or that it's off-limits. Instead, I try to prioritize eating mostly healthy whole foods, and when I really want chocolate, I let myself eat chocolate. A few squares of my favorite bar is almost always how much I need to conquer the craving.

5 **SPLURGING IS NORMAL. IT'S HOW YOU HANDLE A SPLURGE THAT MAKES THE DIFFERENCE BETWEEN FIT AND FAT.** Ever since I started eating mostly whole foods and little processed junk, I rarely overeat. But it can still happen. An occasional binge is actually part of our DNA, left over from the days when humans had to overeat in order to survive long periods without food.

Usually, when I overeat, I can trace the cause. For example, after an all-day photo shoot in Los Angeles recently, I felt irritated, dehydrated, and cold, tired of posing for hours, and I wasn't looking forward to making the trip back to Vail that night. I wanted some sort of reward or treat for enduring all this, and I made the mistake of deciding it should come in the form of food. I stopped on the way to the airport at a frozen yogurt place, where I proceeded to get the largest container of soft-serve possible, which I topped with all sorts of chocolate candies. I ate the whole thing in a matter of minutes, and by the time I got to the airport, I felt sick and awful.

DID YOU KNOW?
Processed Foods Can Make You Depressed

Processed foods aren't just bad for your health; they can also wreak havoc on your happiness. One study found that a diet of mostly processed foods increases the risk of depression by an incredible 58 percent. Eating mostly whole foods, on the other hand, can lower depression risk by 26 percent.

When a binge like this happens to you on occasion, it's normal; what makes the difference is how you recover from it. The first step? Don't beat yourself up. Overeating is never ideal, but it is okay and even natural. You're not a bad person or a pig if you occasionally overdo it with the soft-serve machine, bag of potato chips, or box of cookies.

But try not to do what the majority of people do after a binge: skip your next meal, or give up and decide to keep overeating. Instead, force yourself to eat a small meal or snack with some protein and fat, but no sugar or refined carbs, as soon as possible—eggs scrambled with veggies, plain yogurt or cottage cheese topped with nuts, or a small salad with grilled chicken, olive oil, and vinegar. Even though you're likely not hungry—and the idea of food might even make you nauseous—consuming some sort of a balanced snack is the only way to clear the extra insulin from your blood and stop that vicious sugar-insulin cycle that can trigger overeating hours later.

After my own frozen yogurt splurge, for example, even though the thought of food was sickening, I made myself eat a shrimp salad with avocado at the airport before I flew back. The meal made me feel normal again, countering all that insulin in my blood, which can cause lethargy and cravings. I also know that it helped prevent me from eating something sugary when I got home hours later after a long travel day.

Clean Foods

The following list includes some of my favorite whole foods high in the nutrients that can help your body to burn fat and add muscle. Prioritize the foods on this list when you shop and eat out, but remember, this list is not comprehensive; anything fresh, raw, or that you get out of the ground or straight from a farm or the sea is a great choice. Finally, use your label-reading skills to find those packaged products not listed here that are made mostly from whole-food ingredients.

Avocados

Beans like black, chickpeas, kidney, lentils, lima, and pinto (dry or canned)

Beef and lamb (grass-fed)

Berries like blueberries, cherries, cranberries, raspberries, and strawberries

Bulb vegetables like garlic, leeks, and onions

Citrus fruit like grapefruit, lemons, limes, and oranges

Cruciferous vegetables like broccoli, Brussels sprouts, cabbage, and cauliflower

Cheese

Chicken, duck, and turkey (organic, pasture-raised)

Dark leafy greens like arugula, collard greens, kale, romaine, spinach, and Swiss chard

Eggs (organic, from free-range chickens)

Fermented foods like raw kimchi, sauerkraut, and vinegar

Fish like cod, halibut, salmon, sardines, and tuna

Herbs and spices

Melons like cantaloupe, honeydew, and watermelon

Milk (organic, from grass-fed animals)

Natural sweeteners like honey and maple syrup

Nut butters

Nuts like almonds, cashews, macadamia nuts, and walnuts

Olives and olive oil

Popcorn (stove-top or air-popped)

Pork (organic, pasture-raised)

Root vegetables like beets, carrots, parsnips, radishes, squash, turnips, yams, potatoes, and sweet potatoes

Seeds like chia, hemp, pumpkin, sesame, and sunflower

Shellfish like clams, mussels, oysters, scallops, and shrimp

Vegetables like asparagus, celery, green beans, mushrooms, and tomatoes

Whole grains like barley, brown/wild rice, millet, oats, quinoa, rye, and whole wheat

Whole soy like edamame, miso, tempeh, and tofu (non-GMO, organic)

Yogurt (plain, organic, from grass-fed animals)

Processed Foods and Food Ingredients

The following list details highly processed foods or ingredients found in highly processed foods. While you don't have to totally eliminate all of these items from your diet, you should try to limit consuming them as much as possible. Over time, doing so will lower your cravings for these foods, so much so that the list of clean foods (see opposite) will be much more appealing than the processed stuff, which has been shown to lead to weight gain and poor physical and mental health. Finally, some foods here may be made from whole-food ingredients—be sure to read labels carefully to find them, though.

Added sugars like brown sugar, cane sugar, corn syrup, high-fructose corn syrup, and white sugar

Artificial colors

Artificial flavors

Artificial sweeteners like aspartame, saccharin, and sucralose

Bread crumbs (unless made from 100 percent whole-grain flour, with no additives)

Breakfast cereals (unless made from 100 percent whole-grain ingredients, with no added sugar, preservatives, or other additives)

Brominated vegetable oil (BVO)

Candy

Crackers (unless made from 100 percent whole-grain ingredients, with no added sugars or other additives)

Deli meats that have added nitrates or preservatives or are overly processed

Energy bars (unless made from whole-grain ingredients like nuts, oats, and fruit)

Fast food

Fried food

Frozen yogurt

Fruit juice

Hydrogenated and partially hydrogenated oils like palm and soybean

Ice cream

Jam and jellies

Monosodium glutamate (MSG)

Pita and pita chips (unless made from 100 percent whole-grain ingredients, with no additives)

Potato chips

Preservatives like BHT, BHA, and TBHQ

Pretzels (unless made from 100 percent whole-grain ingredients, with no additives)

Protein powders (unless made from 100 percent whole whey or soy, with no additives)

Refined flours like all-purpose flour, durum wheat flour (in pasta), enriched wheat flour, and white flour

Refined soy like hydrolyzed soy, soy lecithin, and soy protein isolate

Soda

Sodium nitrate and nitrate (typically found in processed meat)

White bread, bagels, buns, cakes, cookies, pies, pizza, pasta, and rice

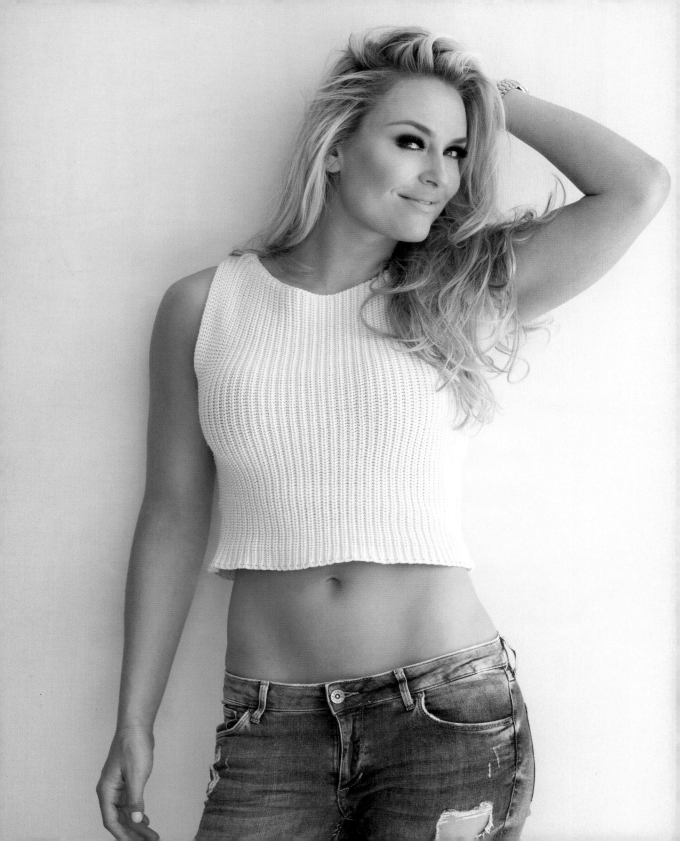

5/
THE ONE-WEEK CHALLENGE

You now know the best way to eat to get strong and lean and the steps you need to take to start. But knowing what to do and actually doing it are two separate things.

Eating mostly fresh or whole foods can be challenging if you've been living on a diet of processed fare for years. But once you get into the habit of eating clean and nourishing your body with healthy, delicious food, I guarantee you'll have so much more energy, be more satisfied, and feel better about your body in general that you won't want to go back to the processed junk again.

Ready to start? Here's how: Commit to eating clean for one week. That's it. That's how long it takes to curb cravings and start feeling leaner and stronger on a program of whole food.

Remember, this is not a diet or a restrictive eating plan that you have to steel yourself to do. Instead, look at it like going on an exciting journey that will expose you to new foods and different ways of consuming them. So pick a day right now—circle it on your calendar or schedule it into your smartphone—and follow these five steps to start your week of eating for a stronger, leaner, healthier, and happier you.

1 CLEAN YOUR KITCHEN. Before you can clean up your diet, it helps to clean out your kitchen. If you're anything like me, I eat what's in my house, meaning that if there's sugary cereal or ice cream around, it is what I'll likely snack on. But if I have to go out and buy these items, it forces me to think twice about whether I really want them—or if I'd be just as satisfied with an apple spread with almond butter. Sometimes the ice cream wins out and I'll get some, but more often than not, I have the apple and am just as satisfied. In other words, out of sight, out of mouth.

To rid your kitchen of junk, get an empty cardboard box and place it in the middle of your kitchen, then use what you learned in chapter 4 about reading ingredients lists. Box up the obvious offenders such as chips, pretzels, cookies, sugary cereals, flavored oatmeal, pastries, refined-flour breads and pasta, frozen meals and pizzas, sugary condiments and sauces, juices (that aren't 100 percent fruit), and soda.

Try to be as discerning as possible. Think of it as a good spring cleaning—your chance to start fresh and begin the week with a clean plate (literally). You'll feel better about getting rid of stuff if you donate the food you don't want to a local food pantry or homeless shelter.

What if you have a husband, kids, or roommates who like the foods you want to get rid of? That's great! No one should be eating processed junk, and you'll be doing everyone a favor by encouraging healthy whole foods over fattening stuff. Remind them that you're not forcing them to undertake some restrictive diet or eating plan but are simply asking them to choose delicious whole foods with real nutritive value over processed stuff for one week. If your partner or roommate needs more convincing, tell them that nutritious food is often more affordable than processed food, especially if you eat out often, as studies show.

2 PLAN YOUR CHALLENGE. Now that the processed junk is gone, it's time to fill your kitchen with delicious, fat-burning foods. But before you hit the farmers' market or grocery store, do a little strategic planning. If you've been living on mostly processed foods for some time, your schedule is likely built around certain ready-to-eat or ready-to-heat meals and snacks. That means it will take a bit of prep work to figure out which simple whole foods are best for your busy schedule and lifestyle.

The day before you begin your one-week challenge, write down exactly what you'll eat for every meal—breakfast, lunch, and dinner—along with two daily snacks for two days total. What to choose? Every meal you plan should include a source of unprocessed protein like fresh chicken, beef, eggs, tofu, or unsweetened dairy, along with a fresh vegetable or fruit, and some fat from whole foods like avocado, olive oil, or nuts. Make sure your meals and snacks also include a starchy carb like oatmeal, quinoa, rice, whole-grain bread, whole-grain pasta, or sweet potatoes. Don't worry about portion size or silly things like the ratio of carbs to protein to fat—right now focus on eating mostly whole foods and little to no processed stuff. Need inspiration? See my favorite meals and snacks in chapter 6.

After you devise a two-day menu, review it with your daily schedule in mind to make sure that you'll have time to prepare all the meals and snacks you listed. For example, if you're used to grabbing a pastry on the way to work (or not eating anything at all), consider choosing a morning meal with no prep time such as a container of plain yogurt with berries and almonds rather than cooked eggs or oatmeal.

The day you start your one-week challenge, remind yourself that you're only locked into your menu for two days. After that, you can plan out the remaining five days, making adjustments based on which meals you enjoy and those that best work with your schedule.

During your first two days, if you start craving a processed snack or something sugary, think of any fresh whole food that will satisfy you instead. When I crave sugar, I'll quash the urge by having a piece of toasted whole-grain bread with butter. Or if I want something savory like chips or crackers, I'll have some crunchy carrots with hummus instead or roasted nuts dusted in ground curry or cumin.

3 **SHOP STRONG.** With your two-day menu in hand, hit the store. Start by shopping for just those things that you'll eat for the next two days, although if you have time to go to the store only once a week, you can do a bigger shop, picking up the whole foods you think you'll enjoy while leaving out the processed stuff.

Here are some tips to help you shop for your one-week challenge:

- Start in the produce section—nearly anything fresh is a good pick for your cart. And don't forget about frozen fruits and vegetables (without any sugary or buttery sauces or preservatives), which can be less expensive than fresh and will last longer.

- Continue shopping the periphery of the store. Stop at the meat department for raw chicken, pork, and beef. Ask for fresh shrimp, tilapia, salmon, and any other fish you like at the seafood counter. Consider canned fish—wild salmon and tuna are good choices—which I've found make convenient and tasty additions to salads and sandwiches. I always pick up eggs, along with plain low-fat dairy like 2% milk, full-fat unsweetened yogurt, and plain cottage cheese. (I prefer low-fat and full-fat dairy, which have less sugar than non-fat varieties and more fat to keep me full.) I don't eat much regular cheese, but if you do, look for those that don't contain any sugar, preservatives, or artificial flavors or colors.

- In the bakery section, use what you learned in chapter 4 to find 100 percent whole-grain bread only. If you can't find one you like at your supermarket, consider going to a natural foods store.

- When you go down the center aisles, be very careful to use everything you learned in chapter 4 to avoid impostor "health" foods. Look for plain quinoa, wild or brown rice, unflavored whole oats (instant, old-fashioned, or steel-cut), and 100 percent whole-grain pasta. If you like beans, go for dried and canned, as long as they don't contain sugar or other additives. Nut butters are great, too—just be sure to check the ingredients list for added sweeteners. Finally, make sure you have some items that aren't sugary to add flavor to your whole foods. I like condiments such as sauerkraut, mustard, and stewed tomatoes, which you can also use for pasta, since most conventional sauces contain added sugar.

- If you don't have it already, invest in a quality cooking oil like olive, expeller-pressed canola, or coconut. A good vinegar like balsamic will also go a long way to help flavor food and makes it easy to whip up a simple junk-free vinaigrette or marinade with olive or coconut oil. I also like to have fresh garlic and ginger on hand, along with plenty of herbs and spices.

4 EAT THREE MEALS AND TWO SNACKS PER DAY. Plenty of diet-book authors and health gurus debate how many meals people should eat to lose weight. As a pro athlete, I get asked the question often, and my answer is always the same: Stop obsessing over it and trying to skip breakfast, or dinner, or go on an intermittent fast—and just start eating three square meals every day, with two small snacks.

I've found—as research shows—that consuming three meals and two snacks daily gives your body the steady supply of calories and nutrients it needs to regulate metabolism, control appetite, prevent cravings, maintain energy, and fuel nonexercise physical activity (meaning you're more likely to opt to take the stairs over the escalator).

If you're not used to eating so often during the day, rethink your habits: Studies show that not eating for hours slows your metabolism

FIVE SECONDS TO A STRONGER YOU
How to Tell Hunger from Craving

Does your body really need food? Or are you just craving the pizza you know is in your fridge? Tell the difference between hunger and craving in an instant by asking yourself, *Am I hungry enough to eat a piece of plain steamed fish?* (Don't like fish? Imagine any plain, unflavored whole food like steamed broccoli or grilled tofu.) If you're really hungry, the idea of eating a whole food will appeal. If not, though, you're probably just having a craving. Curb it by drinking a glass of water or having a cup of tea.

and causes a bigger spike in blood sugar when you do eat, triggering your body to store food more rapidly as fat.

On the other hand, if you think you're saving calories by skipping meals, you're probably not. Research has found that people who don't eat meals end up making up for those calories—and then some—at their next meal. Those who skip meals are also more likely to make poor food choices (like opting for a greasy pizza over a fillet of fish) and to mindlessly snack—like when you sit in front of the TV and suddenly realize you've eaten a whole bag of chips. Knowing that you can eat three meals and two snacks per day also lessens the chance that you'll binge, skip meals when you're hungry, or eat them when you're not.

What if you're not hungry five times a day? Since you should eat only when you're hungry, it will likely take some trial and error for you to figure out what size to make your meals and snacks so that they fill you up while still leaving you hungry in time for the next meal or snack. If you're still not hungry for three square meals, try cutting out one or both daily snacks. Just be sure that you're not making up for either by eating after dinner, when most people are prone to overeat or mindlessly snack.

5 **COOK AT HOME.** When I was in my twenties, I rarely cooked. I didn't know what to make or exactly how to make it and assumed that cooking was a skill that required more time and training than I had, best saved for serious homemakers and professional chefs. Now, though, I know that anyone can cook, even elite athletes who used to think boiling water for spaghetti was a process. More important, making my own meals, especially dinner, has helped transform how I look and feel perhaps more than any other single habit I've discarded.

The thing is, if you don't cook now, it will be difficult for you to

Why You Should Eat Breakfast

I love breakfast—it's my favorite meal of the day. For this reason, I never skip it, a habit that's helped me to get toned and stay lean. Breakfast jump-starts your metabolism in the morning, which triggers your body to start burning calories the minute you get up. The meal also sets the tone for how you'll eat for the rest of the day, meaning if you start by eating healthy, you'll be more likely to keep eating healthy. One study, in fact, found that people who ate eggs for breakfast consumed up to 31 percent fewer calories at lunch than those who skipped the morning meal altogether or had a bowl of sugary cereal.

Eating breakfast also stabilizes low blood sugar—typical if you haven't had any food for 8 to 12 hours—which, in turn, helps prevent cravings later in the day. In fact, research shows that eating breakfast can prevent cravings and overeating for up to 12 hours, meaning that when you eat breakfast, you're less likely to snack after dinner. Finally, breakfast has also been shown to boost alertness, mental function, and even physical performance, helping you get in a better workout if you're a morning exerciser.

If you already eat breakfast, keep it up, but now make sure your morning meal is made up of only low-sugar whole foods. Also be sure to include a good amount of protein and fat, both of which have been shown to jump-start metabolism, right low blood sugar, and keep you feeling full until lunch.

If you don't eat breakfast, I'd encourage you to start—adopting the habit will help you get strong and lean, I promise. For people who aren't used to eating breakfast, it can be something of a shock to the system, so start by having something small like one hard-boiled egg, half a cup of Greek yogurt, or half a piece of whole-grain toast with nut butter. After a few days, you should start to notice a difference: You'll likely have more energy and be less hungry throughout the day. Over time, you'll adjust to eating in the morning and can increase how much you eat.

Eating Whole Can Save You a Whole Lot of Money

Buying healthy whole foods is less expensive than eating out regularly or relying on convenience items like frozen dinners. A recent study found that shopping for fresh foods is 24 percent cheaper per calorie than subsisting on processed stuff.

change your diet enough to change your body: Most prepared, takeout, and restaurant meals are made from processed foods, with double to triple the number of calories of home-cooked fare and up to 50 grams of sugar per meal, according to research. That means that if you're eating prepared meals three times a day, you're consuming a lot of sugar and calories, no matter how nutritious you think your meal is. And even if you're only eating prepared stuff for dinner, it's likely still having a sizable impact on your body, adding at least 16 grams of sugar to your daily intake, according to research.

I get it, I get it: You're busy, and while, sure, you can microwave oatmeal for breakfast and bring a salad to work for lunch, you definitely don't have time to cook dinner. But we're all busy, and if I can find the time to make my own meals, I promise that you can, too. Here's the beautiful thing that I've learned about cooking: Making your own dinner can actually save you time (and money) when you develop an arsenal of quick, easy-to-make meals. There are even studies showing that it takes people the same amount of time to make dinner from fresh ingredients as it does to assemble the meal from prepared foods.

In the next chapter, I share with you some of my favorite go-to dinners, all of which take around twenty minutes to make—about the time it takes to get pizza delivered. This means that even when I'm feeling my laziest (or exhausted from training), I can still get something together without much time or effort.

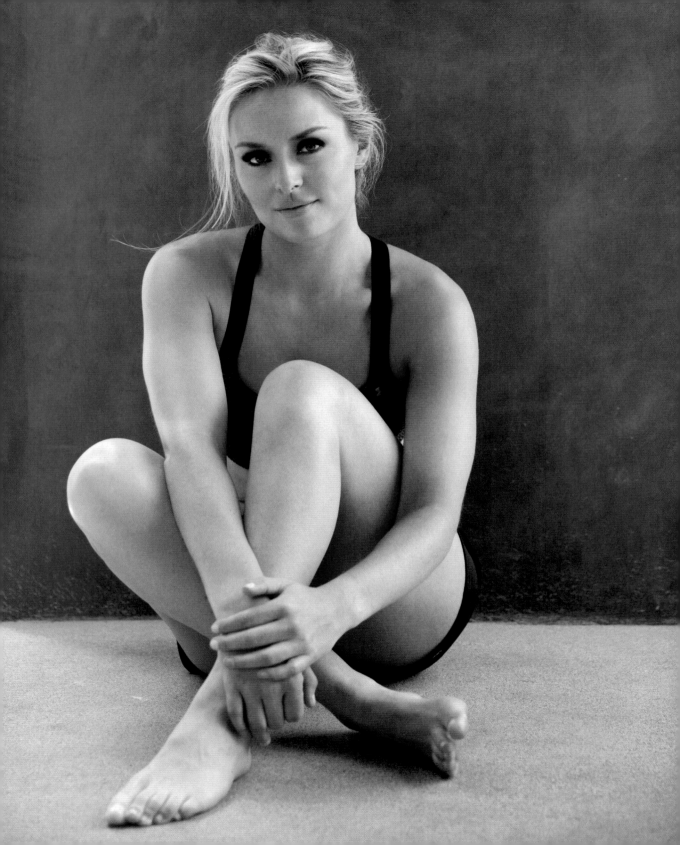

6/ MY FAVORITE GET-STRONG MEALS

like to cook, but I rarely have time to prepare elaborate meals. Sound familiar? If you're like me with a jam-packed schedule, cooking three meals a day is not practical or realistic. But that doesn't mean you have to rely on high-calorie, low-nutrition takeout, ready-to-heat dishes, or processed foods.

Over the years, I've learned that you can still eat healthy home-cooked meals and avoid refined, fattening food by just assembling dishes from fresh ingredients rather than processed ones. One of my favorite meals, for example, is a huge salad with chicken, quinoa, nuts, and avocado, which takes me about five minutes to make. I usually buy a few organic rotisserie chickens when I shop for the week, then slice some of one into a big bowl and warm up the meat briefly in the microwave. Then I'll add fresh spinach, diced avocado, nuts, and some quinoa (which I make in big batches on the weekend), and dress it with olive oil, vinegar, and salt. I give it a good toss, and voilà: Dinner is done.

I also like to make salmon with vegetables, but don't be intimidated by the sound of this. It's one of the fastest meals to make and takes me no more than 15 minutes, start to finish. I'll buy several fillets of wild salmon when I shop for the week, then pan-cook one in olive oil and garlic, which takes a maximum of 10 minutes, depending on the thickness of the fish. At the same time, in a separate pan, I'll sauté fresh green beans in more olive oil and garlic. Then I'll plate both with reheated quinoa or wild rice from the weekend, and I'm ready to eat!

As you can see, cooking doesn't have to be difficult or time-consuming. In fact, it can be faster than relying on takeout or processed meals! In this chapter, you'll find forty-nine of my favorite fast, easy, and simple meals and snacks. Skim this chapter for ideas, but also go online and ask friends for their favorite dishes made with whole foods. I've gleaned many good meal ideas from my friends, some of which I've included here.

FIVE SECONDS TO A STRONGER YOU
Get a Different Plate to Prevent Overeating

On average, we eat 92 percent of the food that we put on our plates, no matter how much we serve ourselves. When I'm eating at home, I use smaller plates and bowls and serve myself a modest amount, since I know that I'll likely consume most of what I put on my plate. When I'm finished, I then assess whether I'm full or need a second helping; most times, I find that I'm totally satisfied. Just don't serve yourself less food on a regular-sized plate: Research shows empty spaces on plates can lead to feelings of deprivation.

Four Tips to Cook Strong

1. **Don't be afraid to experiment with different vegetables** like broccoli rabe, escarole, Swiss chard, rutabaga, parsnips (these make fantastic baked fries, for example), mustard greens, and more. Anything you find fresh in the produce section of the store or at a farmers' market is a whole vegetable and will make a filling addition to any meal.

2. **Think outside the box when it comes to protein.** Wild salmon, tuna, sardines, and anchovies in cans or pouches are fast, easy, and healthy ways to add more protein to your meals. Vegetarian? Try tofu, tempeh, seitan, beans, and nuts. If you're on a budget, organic chicken thighs are cheap and contain more minerals and healthy fat than chicken breasts. If you like red meat, experiment with elk, bison, or venison, all of which are usually pasture-raised, making for healthier cuts of meat.

3. **Yes, you can eat breakfast for dinner**—or lunch for breakfast, dinner for lunch, and so on. Breakfast is my favorite meal, so why not have it twice a day? Oftentimes my lunch and dinner salads are interchangeable, although I often eat more carbs at lunch, meaning I'll add quinoa to my salad in the afternoon but not at night. Again, it's all about finding the balance that gives you the most energy and makes you feel full.

4. **What to do about snacks?** All my grab-and-go suggestions for breakfast and lunch make ideal snacks, too.

BREAKFAST

GRAB AND GO

Grab at least two of the following and go:

Container of plain Greek yogurt (add fruit and/or nuts)

Banana or apple with packet of nut butter

Pre-portioned bag of nuts

Hard-boiled eggs

Microwaved eggs (scrambled eggs microwaved in a mug for several minutes)

String cheese with an apple and whole-grain crispbread

Packet of instant unflavored oatmeal mixed with touch of honey or maple syrup

Egg muffins

Make on the weekend to grab and go during the week: In a large bowl, combine eggs, chopped spinach, broccoli, onion, bell peppers, mushrooms, tomatoes, or other veggies of choice. Add a splash of milk and a small amount of shredded or crumbled fresh cheese if desired. Season with salt, pepper, and/or herbs and spices like dried basil, dill, and red pepper flakes. Pour into cups of a muffin tin and bake at 350°F until brown and the eggs are set, 10 to 20 minutes. Wrap individual muffins, refrigerate, then grab and go!

Baked oatmeal

Make on the weekend to grab and go during the week: In a large bowl, combine 2 cups oatmeal with milk, cinnamon, and a touch of maple syrup. Add berries or sliced banana for more flavor, or omit syrup and add shredded zucchini or carrot for more fiber. You can also add crushed nuts, an egg, and/or nut butter for extra flavor, fat, and protein. Pour into a pan and bake at 350°F until center is set, about 30 minutes. Cut into squares, cover pan, and refrigerate. Heat briefly before grabbing and going.

EGGS

Lindsey's go-to egg scramble

Sauté onions, peppers, and mushrooms in olive oil until soft. Add eggs and scramble. Top with diced avocado, salsa, and fresh cilantro. Enjoy with whole-grain toast with almond butter.

Veggie scramble

Sauté baby spinach, red pepper, broccoli, onion, tomato, or other fresh veggies in olive oil until wilted or soft. Add eggs and scramble. Season with fresh basil, red pepper flakes, hot sauce, or other herbs or spices.

Easy eggs Benedict

Cook one slice of pancetta, Canadian bacon, or dry-cured bacon. Poach an egg. Place egg and bacon on piece of whole-grain toast, and top with Greek yogurt mixed with mustard and a touch of lemon juice for a healthier homemade hollandaise.

OATMEAL

Lindsey's go-to oatmeal

Cook steel-cut oats. Top with honey (preferably raw, which is less processed, or locally sourced) and nuts. Consider adding an extra source of protein like eggs or yogurt.

Banana bread oatmeal

Cook steel-cut, traditional, or instant unflavored oatmeal. When set, stir in banana, chopped nuts, and a touch of maple syrup. Consider adding an extra source of protein like eggs or yogurt.

Savory oatmeal bowl

Cook steel-cut, traditional, or instant unflavored oatmeal. Fold in sautéed mushrooms, garlic, and thyme, or top with a fried egg, sriracha, scallions, and crushed peanuts. Or try making oatmeal with tomato puree and add fresh basil and a touch of Parmesan cheese once cooked. Consider adding an extra source of protein like eggs or yogurt if your bowl doesn't include it.

Sweet potato oatmeal

Cook steel-cut, traditional, or instant unflavored oatmeal. Stir in mashed sweet potato and top with chopped pecans, cinnamon, and a touch of maple syrup. Consider adding an extra source of protein like eggs or yogurt.

YOGURT

Apple- or berry-pie parfait

Mix plain Greek yogurt with a touch of cinnamon. Layer or mix with sliced apples or berries and crushed walnuts or sliced almonds. Add toasted rolled oats or low-sugar whole-grain granola if desired.

Savory yogurt bowl

Mix plain Greek yogurt in a bowl with roasted veggies, sautéed garlic, and a drizzle of olive oil. Or try mixing in chopped nuts or seeds with chopped olives and spices like cumin, curry powder, or even harissa paste.

PB and Y

Swirl nut butter of choice into plain unflavored yogurt and top with fresh strawberries, raspberries, and/or blueberries. Top with chopped nuts for crunch.

SANDWICHES

Breakfast burrito

Scramble eggs with black beans. Place inside a warm whole-grain tortilla; add sliced avocado and salsa. Sprinkle with shredded cheese or top with a dollop of Greek yogurt.

Egg-bacon muffin

Cook one slice of pancetta, dry-cured bacon, or Canadian bacon, then use the same pan to cook an egg until soft and runny. Place egg and bacon on one slice of whole-grain English muffin or toast; top with sliced fresh tomato. Spread mashed avocado on a second piece of whole-grain muffin or toast, and top to make a sandwich.

Salmon toast

On whole-grain bread, English muffin, or crispbread, smear some goat cheese, feta, ricotta, thick Greek yogurt mixed with salt and herbs, or other healthy whole-food spread. Top with smoked salmon.

Avocado toast

Spread mashed avocado on whole-grain toast. Top with a sunny-side-up egg, diced tomato and fresh basil, crushed almonds or pistachios, or just sea salt and pepper. The combinations are endless.

PB&S quesadilla

Spread a whole-grain tortilla with peanut butter; top with sliced banana and strawberry. Fold in half and panfry with a touch of olive oil on both sides until lightly browned.

INDULGENCES

My favorite French toast

Combine egg, milk, cinnamon, and nutmeg in dish. Toast pieces of whole-grain bread, then dip into egg mixture and panfry with a touch of butter. Spread toast with nut butter, butter, or a touch of maple syrup. Pair with a source of protein like eggs or yogurt.

Vanessa's protein pancakes

In a blender, blend 1 egg, 1/2 cup oat flour, and 1 ripe banana until well combined. Cook as you would classic pancakes. Top with grass-fed butter or coconut butter. No syrup necessary!

Classic whole-grain pancakes

Substitute whole wheat or whole-grain gluten-free flour for all-purpose or white flour in your favorite homemade pancake recipe. Top with nut butter or fresh fruit instead of maple syrup to reduce sugar load (or use maple syrup sparingly). For a savory take, fold in cooked and shredded broccoli, zucchini, carrots, butternut or winter squash, or sweet potato; season with cumin, salt, pepper, and/or other herbs and spices. Pair with a source of protein like eggs or yogurt.

Sweet potato breakfast bake

Bake a sweet potato until soft. Cut in half and top with chopped nuts, raisins, cinnamon, and a drizzle of honey or a dollop of yogurt. Pair with a source of protein like eggs or yogurt.

LINDSEY'S LESSONS
Slow Down to Get Strong

Growing up in a large family, I learned to eat meals quickly—if I didn't, I never got seconds! But when you consume food too quickly, it's almost impossible to tell when you're full, which means you're likely to end up eating more without noticing or even enjoying it. Studies show that fast eaters consume more than 3 ounces of food per minute than slower eaters. Learn to take your time by chewing each mouthful completely before swallowing and putting down your fork between bites. Focus on how each forkful or handful of food tastes before reaching for more.

LUNCH

GRAB AND GO

Grab three of the following and go:

Single-serving container of roasted chicken, grilled steak, shrimp, tuna, tofu, etc.

Single-serving container of quinoa, brown rice, wild rice, barley, etc.

Bag of organic beef or chicken jerky (check the label for sugar)

String cheese or cubed cheese with fruit or veggies

Plain Greek yogurt (add fruit and/ or nuts)

Hard-boiled eggs

Pre-portioned bag of carrots, cherry tomatoes, broccoli, cucumbers, etc.

Carrots, bell peppers, or cucumbers with a small container of hummus

Apple, pear, or banana with a packet of nut butter

Pre-portioned bag of nuts

Pre-portioned bag of air-popped popcorn

Celery topped with nut butter and raisins

SALADS

Lindsey's go-to salad

Top baby spinach with cooked quinoa, sliced chicken from a rotisserie chicken, berries, and a handful of chopped mixed nuts. Dress with vinaigrette.

Strawberry chicken

Top mixed greens or arugula with sliced roasted chicken, strawberries, red onion, cooked wheat berries, walnuts, and goat cheese. Dress with vinaigrette.

Simple Greek
Top romaine with grilled chicken or shrimp, tomatoes, black or green olives, chickpeas, pine nuts, and feta cheese. Dress with vinaigrette.

Shrimp endive
Top endive with steamed shrimp, sliced apple or pear, walnuts, crumbled blue cheese, and toasted, cubed whole-grain bread. Dress with vinaigrette.

Wild rice with cherries and pork
Top baby kale, Swiss chard, or mustard greens with sliced pork tenderloin or chicken sausage, wild rice, cherries or other berries, sliced almonds, and Parmesan. Dress with vinaigrette.

Southwestern steak
Top romaine or mixed greens with grilled steak, corn, black beans, roasted red peppers, and avocado. Dress with vinaigrette.

Winter vegetarian salad
Top baby kale with cubed grilled tofu, cubed baked sweet potato, cooked barley, pistachios, and pomegranate arils. Dress with vinaigrette.

Salmon or tuna Niçoise
Top romaine with canned wild salmon or light tuna, green beans, cubed cooked potatoes, black olives, and cherry tomatoes. Dress with vinaigrette.

Simple Thai
Top mixed greens with whole-grain soba noodles, grilled chicken, shrimp, or tofu, julienned carrots, sliced red bell pepper, bean sprouts, and crushed nuts or sesame seeds. Dress with a vinaigrette made from nut butter mixed with lime juice and soy sauce.

Salmon pasta salad

Cook whole-grain fusilli when you have time. Mix with canned wild salmon or light tuna, arugula or baby spinach, and chopped red bell peppers, tomatoes, or sun-dried tomatoes. Dress with olive oil and red-wine vinegar, and top with shaved Parmesan.

SANDWICHES

Healthy BLT

Spread toasted whole-grain bread lightly with olive oil. Top with lettuce, sliced tomato, and dry-cured organic bacon. Top with a dollop of plain tuna fish, crabmeat, or cooked shrimp for more protein.

PB and fruit

Spread whole-grain bread with nut butter. Top with sliced apples, banana, and/or strawberries or raspberries. You can also use an all-fruit spread with no sugar added, but fresh fruit is better.

Bread-free Italian sandwich

Grill two portobello mushrooms or two thick slices of eggplant when you have time, and refrigerate. When you're ready to make a sandwich, remove mushrooms or eggplant slices from fridge, top with fresh mozzarella, and heat in a pan or in the microwave. Add sliced tomato and fresh basil. Or top either with a poached egg, dry-cured or Canadian bacon, tomato, and avocado.

Middle Eastern wrap

Spread a whole-grain tortilla or whole-grain pita with hummus. Fill with baby spinach, chopped cucumber, sliced red onion, chopped hard-boiled egg, and avocado.

Easy egg salad

Mix chopped hard-boiled eggs with Greek yogurt or organic mayo (most mayonnaise contains sugar and other highly processed ingredients, so read labels carefully), mustard, and chives. Spread on whole-grain bread or use to fill a whole-grain pita; top with lettuce, tomato, and onion. You can also serve this over spinach or mixed greens.

Easy chicken salad

Mix chopped cooked chicken with Greek yogurt or organic mayo (see note in egg salad), touch curry powder, sliced grapes, and chopped nuts. Spread on whole-grain bread or use to fill a whole-grain pita; top with lettuce, tomato, and onion. You can also serve this over spinach or mixed greens.

Chicken, cheddar, and grapes

Spread whole-grain bread with olive oil. Top with a slice of cheddar or Swiss cheese. Panfry until cheese melts. Remove from heat, add sliced grapes or strawberries, and top with lettuce or baby spinach.

Pizza sandwich

Toast a whole-grain English muffin. Top with tomato puree or sugar-free tomato sauce (read labels carefully) and shredded cheese. Pair with a protein like roasted chicken, grilled steak, or shrimp.

DID YOU KNOW?
Why Dining Out Can Be a Disaster

The average restaurant meal contains 1,128 calories—more than half the recommended daily 2,000-calorie intake for active women.

DINNER

Lindsey's go-to dinner

Panfry salmon in olive oil and minced garlic. Serve with cooked quinoa and grilled or panfried asparagus in olive oil.

Clean and lean burger with fries

Cut sweet potatoes into spears and brush with olive oil; season with salt and pepper and other spices or herbs. Bake in single layer on sheet pan at 450°F until tender and golden, about 20 minutes. Shape 90 percent lean ground bison, turkey, or burger meat into patties; season and grill or panfry until done. Serve on whole-grain bread or wrapped in a sturdy piece of lettuce alongside a steamed vegetable.

Good-for-you pasta with meatballs

Mix ground sirloin, turkey, or chicken with an egg, chopped onion, minced garlic, Worcestershire sauce, and herbs and spices like oregano, basil, and parsley. Shape into meatballs and bake in the oven at 350°F until done. Cook whole-grain pasta. Mix with olive oil and fresh chopped tomatoes, tomato puree, or sugar-free pasta sauce (read labels carefully). Top with meatballs and shaved Parmesan.

Lemon-caper chicken or fish

Panfry chicken or a healthy fish like salmon or halibut in olive oil and minced garlic. Remove protein, then add lemon juice, wine, and drained capers. Bring to a boil and add a touch of butter and whole wheat flour if desired to thicken. Cook and serve over protein with roasted potatoes and spinach sautéed in olive oil.

Healthy "fried" rice

Cook brown or wild rice until done. In a skillet, sauté chopped onion and garlic in olive oil. Add peas and carrots (thawed if frozen) and cook until warm. Add rice and cook until warm, adding more oil to pan if needed; season with salt, pepper, and spice. While stirring, add one or two beaten eggs, and cook for several minutes, stirring, until egg coats rice mixture. You can also add chopped cooked chicken, shrimp, pork tenderloin, or black beans for more protein before adding eggs.

Easy stuffed squash

Halve an acorn or delicata squash and remove seeds. Brush the insides with olive oil and salt, and roast at 425°F until soft, about 30 minutes. In a skillet, sauté chopped onion and garlic; add ground sirloin, chicken, or turkey; season with salt, pepper, and chili powder; and cook until done. Stir in cooked quinoa, barley, or wild rice, and heat until warm. Remove from heat and use to fill roasted squash halves. Top stuffed squash with toasted pepitas or pumpkin seeds, crumbled queso fresco, or a dollop of plain Greek yogurt. You can also experiment with stuffing with a quinoa or rice mixture that includes dried fruit, nuts, and chicken, or sautéed chicken sausage and torn kale.

Frittata with salad

In large bowl, whisk eggs. Add any fresh greens like baby spinach, arugula, and kale, and/or add slightly sautéed veggies like broccoli, onions, bell peppers, asparagus, mushrooms, leeks, or cubed potatoes. Season with salt, pepper, and herbs or spices, and add a touch of milk. You can also add smoked salmon, cooked pancetta or bacon, or a touch of cheese for more protein. Pour egg mixture into an oven-safe pan and heat over medium-low heat until eggs set, only several minutes. Transfer to oven and broil until top is lightly browned. Serve with side salad.

Healthy pizza

Substitute whole wheat flour in your favorite homemade pizza dough recipe or buy a premade 100 percent whole wheat pizza crust (read label carefully for added sugar and to make sure it's 100 percent whole grains).

Spread with pesto, tomato puree, tomato sauce (read label carefully for added sugar), or mashed avocado. Top with shredded or crumbled fresh cheese and any vegetable you'd like, including spinach, kale, escarole, broccoli, broccoli rabe, sliced onion, corn—the sky's the limit. Season with herbs like basil, oregano, or thyme. Bake according to instructions. For more protein, add grilled chicken, shrimp, crumbled pancetta, crumbled chicken sausage, or fried egg.

Easy Sunday stew with whole-grain croutons
In a large pot, sauté lean steak (or substitute chicken thighs or tofu). Remove from pot and cut meat into bite-size pieces. Sauté chopped onion, garlic, and carrots. Lower the heat and add tomato paste (to thicken and impart flavor), along with any vegetables of choice (thaw if frozen) like broccoli, cauliflower, kale, mushrooms, peas, corn, asparagus tips, cubed sweet or white potatoes, or asparagus. Add meat back to the pot and enough low-sodium beef or chicken broth to cover ingredients. Season with salt, pepper, rosemary, thyme, paprika, bay leaves, a splash of wine or whiskey, and/or other seasonings of choice. Cook over low heat for several hours. Refrigerate for up to one week. Serve with toasted, cubed whole-grain bread brushed with olive oil and salt, or over brown or wild rice.

DESSERT

J's favorite protein balls
In the bowl of a food processor, mix one 15.5-ounce can chickpeas (rinsed and drained), $\frac{1}{2}$ cup almond meal, $\frac{1}{4}$ cup unsweetened peanut butter, $\frac{3}{4}$ cup honey, $\frac{3}{4}$ teaspoon vanilla extract, 2 tablespoons chia seeds, and $\frac{1}{2}$ cup dark chocolate chips until smooth. Roll into 24 bite-sized balls, place on foil-lined pan, and freeze until firm.

FITNESS

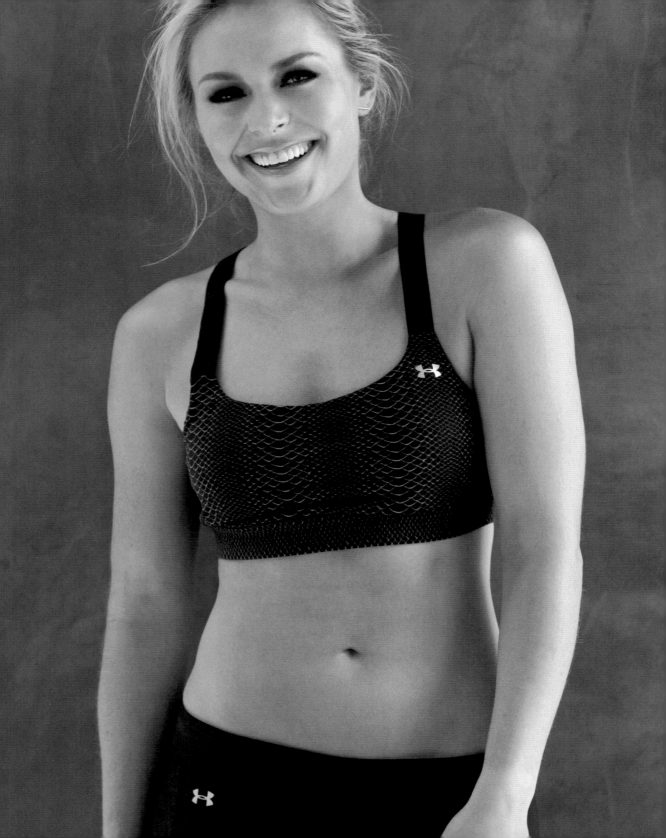

7/ FINDING YOUR FITNESS YOU

have a confession to make: I hate running. Or let's just say that I strongly dislike it and never do it. Running in gym class as a kid, I loathed every minute—my knees hurt, it made my hips sore, I felt uncoordinated, and there was no point ever when I didn't wish I was playing any other sport. When my father started taking me to the track to help me get in shape for the ski team, I still didn't like running, but I was willing to do it to pass the test in order to make the U.S. ski team.

When I look back at my younger self, though, I wonder what would have happened if I hadn't found skiing and I'd only tried jogging or sports that include a lot of running. I would still be in sports in some capacity, but I'm not sure that I'd be a professional athlete.

The possibility that I might not be a professional athlete is difficult to even consider because—and here's my second confession—I love training. I'm not exaggerating; I really enjoy working out. If I had to stop skiing tomorrow, I'd still exercise almost every day only because I love it so much and I've seen how training has changed my life in so many positive ways that I couldn't even imagine who I'd be—and who I'd become—without it.

Working out has helped me win medals and world records, of course, but it's also turned a girl from Minnesota with insecurities just like everyone else's into a confident woman. Exercise has helped give me the courage to chase my dreams and keep chasing them no matter the setbacks or serious injury life throws me. It's made me more determined, not only to get the most out of my sport but also to get the most out of my life.

I realize that most people don't love working out, and many have to force themselves to exercise—if they even exercise at all. That makes me sad, because I believe everyone would love working out as much as I do if they only took the time and the effort to find activities that make them truly happy. I wasn't born with some elusive gene that makes me love working out, after all—no one is. It wasn't until I found my Fitness Me—or who I am in the gym and on the hill—that I developed the passion for working out that I have today.

That's a big reason why I wanted to write this book: to help you find your Fitness You, or the way of working out that will make you your happiest and healthiest. We all go on a journey through life to find ourselves as individuals, and finding your Fitness You—how you best express yourself through activity, exercise, or movement—is no different. It takes time and effort. You may have to try a dozen different machines, sports outside the gym, or even those activities that aren't traditionally perceived as exercise until you discover something that you truly enjoy. But at the end of the journey to find your Fitness You, you'll want to exercise just as much as you like to do any hobby, and it'll be second nature to do exactly what your body needs to be strong and lean.

How I Found My Fitness Me

I fell in love with skiing at a very young age, but that doesn't mean I found my Fitness Me when I was two—that'd be similar to someone saying that she found what makes her happy for life at age two. It took time to learn what I truly enjoy and what I could do often enough to make me happy.

When I was a kid, I threw myself into every activity that I could—fairly easy to do when you have four siblings. I biked, swam, and hiked in the summers, and sledded and skied in the winters. Out of school, I played soccer, gymnastics, and took figure skating lessons.

While I liked many of these activities and sports, none was as fun as skiing, particularly racing. I liked the feeling of going fast and pushing myself to go faster, and I connected better with the kids who raced than with those who did gymnastics or skated. No one ever forced me to ski—it was always what I wanted to do. And it made me happy.

By the time I was nine, after I met Olympic skier Picabo Street, I knew that I wanted to race professionally. But I had to make the U.S. Ski Team first, which meant passing a rigorous fitness test. When I was fourteen, I began working with a trainer and lifting weights, and my father starting taking me to the track to run at night and on the weekends.

I didn't enjoy lifting as a teenager, and I hated running. Thankfully, though, I was determined to find another way to get the aerobic activity I needed, and that's how I discovered cycling. I got a bike and starting doing long rides down the roads near my childhood home in Minnesota and through the mountain valleys of Vail. I loved it. It didn't make my body hurt like running, and I could challenge myself on the bike in a way I was never able to on the track, testing myself to climb Vail Pass without stopping or bike the thirty miles to a Minnesota lake in less time than I did the week prior.

This was a critical discovery for me as an athlete because I realized that to enjoy a workout, I needed a way to challenge myself to go longer, harder, faster, or farther. Not everyone is competitive or likes to be when they exercise, but I am, and discovering that I enjoy an inherent challenge when working out has helped me create routines that are more satisfying and rewarding. Today I still prefer to bike for

DID YOU KNOW?

80 Percent of People Are Missing Out on More Joy

Only 20 percent of Americans meet the federal criteria for getting enough physical and muscle-strengthening activity on a weekly basis, according to statistics.

aerobic exercise, and I've found new rides and ways to challenge my-self while training in Europe and all over the world, as well as around my home in Vail.

I love lifting weights now, but I didn't enjoy strength training at first. It took time to develop the confidence that I needed to feel good about working out in the weight room and to find the exercises that made me feel mentally and physically strong. This meant experimenting with many different routines and ways of strengthening my body before I found what I love and am addicted to doing.

Even though I began skiing professionally at fifteen, I've never stopped trying new sports and ways of working out. After all, you never stop growing and finding yourself as a person, so why would you ever end the adventure of finding your Fitness You?

Today I'm always watching what other athletes and people do in the gym to try to find new ways to train. People are constantly coming up with clever, creative workouts to get strong, and I believe that you can learn from anyone, no matter their sport, fitness ability, or experience level. And that's another thing I love about working out—you can find inspiration everywhere you look.

All the Ways I Love to Work Out

If I weren't a skier, I might have played tennis competitively—or at least tried, as I'm not very good at it. But I love the game—it's challenging, a fantastic workout, and a great way to get out aggression. Before my first knee injury, I played frequently, hitting off a ball machine whenever I was in Florida. While I can't play now because I'm worried I'll reinjure my knee, I plan to play again after I retire from skiing and don't have to be as concerned about further damage.

Over the years, there are many other sports I've discovered I enjoy doing, and today I love spending my off-seasons experimenting with as many as I can while regularly doing the ones that can help me ski better. Here are some of my favorite ways to work out off the hill.

Weight lifting	Golf	Free diving
Bodyweight training	Slacklining	Spearfishing
Plyometric training	Dancing	Stand up paddle boarding
Elliptical	Canoeing	Spin class
Road cycling	Volleyball	Squash
Spinning	Hiking	Boxing
Tennis	Walking my dogs	
Horseback riding	Fly-fishing	

Finding Your Fitness You

If you think you've tried enough ways of working out to know categorically that exercise is not fun, let me tell you a story: I started skiing when I was two, and since then, I've tried dozens of different sports. Spearfishing! Horseback riding! Gymnastics! Soccer! Even fly-fishing and diving for lobsters! Still, after spending hours in the gym every day for the past fifteen-plus years and working out with all kinds of coaches and athletes doing innovative exercises, I can't say that I've tried every way of working out to get strong and lean.

In reality, few people experiment with exercise. They try a few machines at the gym, maybe a couple of weight-lifting moves, and perhaps several sports like running, tennis, or swimming. But when it comes to all the ways you could possibly move your body to tone up or lean down, using a few gym machines or playing a sport or two are just a small glimpse into the great wide world of fitness.

Think about it: Have you really played tennis since you were a kid or tried swimming regularly for fitness in a pool? How many weight-lifting exercises have you done more than a handful of times? And have you really considered all the dozens of gym machines, cardio classes, strength-training exercises, dance forms, yoga styles, boot camps, outdoor games, winter sports, summer sports, gardening, and all other ways to move your body that can make you strong and lean? There's a big, exciting world of physical fitness out there just waiting for you, so get ready and start the journey today to find your Fitness You.

Five Steps to Find Your Fitness You

1   MAKE A LIST OF ALL THE POSSIBLE ACTIVITIES YOU THINK YOU MIGHT EVER ENJOY. Get a piece of paper and write down every physical activity you enjoy now or think you might enjoy—gardening, hiking, kayaking, learning to salsa dance, training for a 5K, doing the elliptical, weight lifting, taking a Spin class, or trying a pole-dancing class.

If you belong to a gym or like the idea of working out in a gym, write down exercises, classes, and machines that you know about, but also try to think of things you might enjoy outside the gym. If you don't like the gym and have actually tried it—meaning you've spent enough time at several different locations, as gyms can vary hugely in offerings and overall vibe—that's totally fine. There are many things you can do without ever setting foot inside a gym, including the exercises of my nine circuit workouts on pages 165 to 229.

2 TRY AT LEAST ONE NEW WORKOUT FOR TWENTY MINUTES EVERY WEEK. Make it your goal to try at least one new workout every week for one month. Keep an open mind, but don't feel pressured to like whatever you try right away—you probably won't. Your purpose right now is simply to explore and find what you think you might want to try again.

There's just one rule: You can't count something as "trying it" if you do a workout for only five minutes—that's not long enough to give your body time to warm up, let alone adapt to the movements you're doing. Try to sustain any cardio-based workout for twenty minutes, easing into the exercise at first by going slower than you think you should. If you're trying new strengthening exercises or lifting weights, warm up your muscles beforehand by walking or riding a bike for at least five minutes, then rotate through different sets, or exercises, for ten to fifteen minutes.

3 **IF YOU GIVE SOMETHING FIVE STARS OUT OF TEN, TRY IT AGAIN NEXT WEEK.** But if you dislike something, cross it off the list. Just know that you're probably not going to fall in love with a new workout right away. So if something seems even remotely interesting, circle a date on your calendar the following week to try it again. It doesn't matter why you like it—maybe you think the StairMaster makes your butt look better or you spotted a cute guy in a vinyasa yoga class. Those are reasons enough to try it again. On the other hand, if something made your body hurt or you just weren't enjoying yourself after twenty minutes, you don't have to try it again. The goal here is to find one or two exercises that you enjoy—and it's icing on the cake if you discover more.

4 **FOUR IS THE MAGIC NUMBER.** Try any workouts that you think you might like at least four times before deciding if they're a good fit for you. Four sessions should be enough to determine whether a workout has the potential to positively affect your body and mood.

If you find something you enjoy, congratulations! In the next chapter, I'll show you how to make this exercise part of your weekly or daily routine.

If nothing excites you, though, that's okay. Sit down again to make a new list—and this time, get more creative. Think outside the gym to outdoor sports, athletic clubs, adult pickup games, and dance classes that you might enjoy. Or if you like the idea of exercising at the gym but still haven't found something you like to do there, consider looking for a new gym with different class offerings, machines, or even atmosphere. I know some people who don't like to work out at gyms without personal TVs or those that don't have any windows near the cardio equipment.

5 **KEEP THE ADVENTURE ALIVE.** Once you find a workout you enjoy, keep the spirit of adventure alive because exercise, no matter how much you like it, can get monotonous and boring at times. It's a lot like food, in fact: If you had to eat the same meal every day, even if it was your favorite meal, wouldn't you eventually get sick of it and want to try something different? Continually experimenting as you find your Fitness You will keep your workouts fresh, help you stay motivated, and challenge your body in new ways so that you continue to get strong and lean without ever getting stuck in a rut.

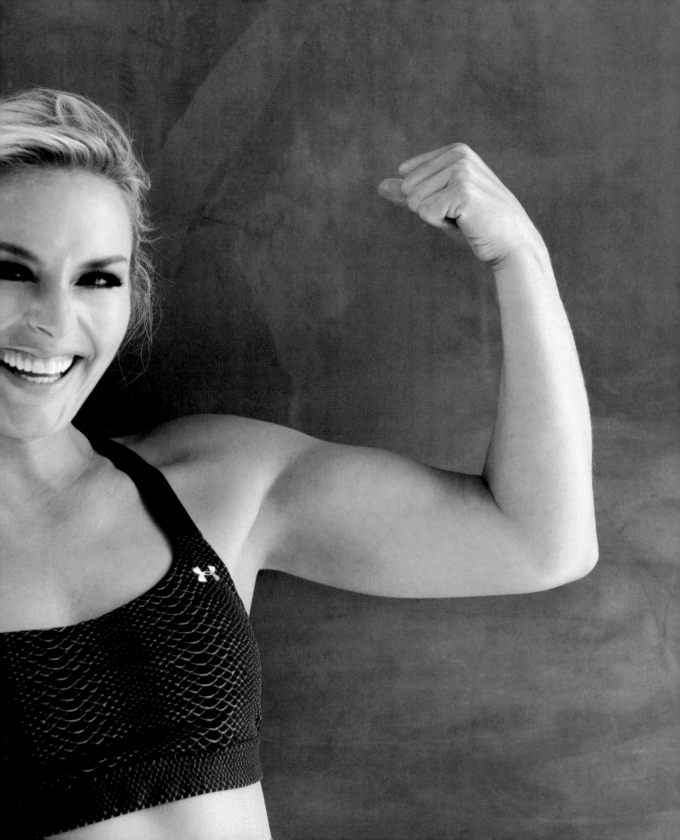

8/ NINE WAYS TO MAKE EXERCISE A HAPPY HABIT

During the winter months when I'm racing, I wake up at five-thirty in the morning so that I can work out before I ski. To anyone who knows me well, this is a labor of love, because I relish my sleep—and usually, wherever I am in Europe, it's cold, dark, and fairly unfriendly at five-thirty in the morning. But I've learned that waking up early is a small price to pay to do the things I need to do on a regular basis to improve my body in momentous ways.

The thing is, if you want to change your body and your health, you will likely have to make small changes to your daily routine, too. These changes, while minor, are still challenging—it's part of human nature, after all, to prefer consistency, and anything that upsets our sense of routine and "normal" will likely make us uncomfortable at first. But the only way to become successful at anything, whether it's playing a sport, learning a new skill, or reshaping your body, is to make small daily changes and sustain these changes until they become part of a new routine—your new "normal." This doesn't mean doing something differently for one day here or there, but trying to establish a new habit that becomes part of your regular routine.

The good news, though, is that once you make a small change to your routine, you may come to enjoy or even prefer it. And when you start to see results from your new routine as your body gets stronger and leaner, I promise you'll never want to give up your old habits.

So how exactly do you change your daily routine so that working out becomes a normal and enjoyable part of your life? Here are the nine ways I've found to get hooked on the exercise habit.

1 STOP USING THE ONE EXCUSE THAT WILL PREVENT YOU FROM GETTING STRONG AND LEAN. Think you don't have time to work out on a weekly basis—or exercise at all? The first step to making exercise part of your life is to stop deluding yourself with this weak excuse. Because if you spend *any* time watching TV, catching up on social media, or surfing the web like most people do for hours every day, guess what? You have time to exercise.

In fact, 96 percent of all Americans enjoy several hours of daily leisure time, most of which they use watching TV for an average of 2.8 hours per day. That's almost three hours of sitting on your rump, staring at colored pixels! Even if you hit the gym for an hour every day, you'd still have nearly two hours left to catch your favorite shows. Plus, you could always do what I do: Catch your favorite specials while pedaling the indoor bike—more on that on page 126.

2 FIND A TIME TO EXERCISE, THEN HIT REPEAT. Sit down with your daily or weekly calendar and think about the most practical time of day you can exercise at least three days per week. Is it easier for you to work out first thing in the morning so that if projects come up at work or you have social events at night, you don't have to choose between exercise and these activities? Or would you enjoy the stress relief and pre-dinner routine that working out at night can provide?

No matter when you exercise, building in consistent workout slots on your weekly calendar makes it more likely that you'll exercise than if you choose to wake up every day and wonder if and when you should go to the gym. Scheduling your workout time helps make exercise as much part of your routine as your daily shower or office meetings: No matter the week or what comes up, you always know that at X o'clock on A, B, and C days, you'll be at the gym, just as at Y o'clock during your workweek, you're always in the shower.

3 **THINK PRACTICAL, NOT PIPE DREAM.** Setting a challenge for your-self like running a 5K in a certain time, finishing a sprint-distance triath-lon, or simply getting to the gym three days a week can help motivate you to exercise on a regular basis—that is, *if* your goal is realistic to your current lifestyle and fitness level. Otherwise, an unrealistic goal can backfire and make it less likely that you'll continue to work out.

For example, if you tell yourself that you're going to exercise for an hour every day when you haven't worked out for more than ten minutes total in months, you're likely setting a goal you won't be able to sustain. Instead, consider a more feasible challenge like walking outside for twenty to thirty minutes every other day. Achieving a realistic goal and feeling that sense of accomplishment when you do will help transform your body more than setting an impractical but more challenging goal that it's unlikely you can meet.

Even as a pro athlete, I've learned to readjust my daily goals when I realize that something I told myself I can or should do is not realistic. For example, if I'm scheduled to do a long or difficult workout on a day that I suddenly have a multi-hour photo shoot, I'll push that challeng-ing workout to later in the week and do something easier or shorter instead. This way, I prevent not only the likelihood of a bad workout because I was too tired or stressed to give it my all, but also the possi-bility of feeling like a failure because it was highly unlikely that I would meet my original goal.

4 **IT'S NOT THAT HARD—OR AT LEAST, IT DOESN'T HAVE TO BE.** You don't need to fall over in exhaustion or throw up after a workout to tone up and get lean. In fact, if you push yourself too hard every time you exercise, you're more likely to get injured and not be able to tone at all. Worse still, you can also start loathing a workout that you once loved.

Whether it's a fifteen-minute-per-mile walk or a five-minute-per-mile sprint, simply moving your body more will help you get strong and lean. In fact, studies show that standing or walking for longer periods of time than you're used to can lower blood sugar and improve insulin levels better than super-intense exercise, which can be jarring to your body and metabolic system.

Of course, if you enjoy pushing yourself and already have some base fitness, it's perfectly fine to do a hard or long workout once or twice a week. But if you're not a glutton for punishment, don't feel like you have to undertake a grueling exercise program or hire a trainer who leaves you in tears at the end of every workout.

While high-intensity training has many benefits, it also has one considerable detriment: It drains your willpower. Willpower works like a muscle: Use it too often and you'll tire it out. If you're continually forcing yourself to do a strenuous workout several times a week, it can exhaust your inclination to adopt other healthy habits, like eating right. In fact, research shows that people who work out intensely often make poorer food decisions than those who don't because they literally exhaust their willpower to eat healthy.

5 **EMBRACE THE MINI-GOAL.** I set goals for everything, not just for my workouts but also for what I want to accomplish today, tomorrow, this year, and even in my lifetime.

I've already talked about how setting realistic goals can help motivate you to work out—the same is true about having goals you can attain more quickly than others. If you're like me and are inspired by challenges, setting daily or weekly mini-goals can help you stay motivated to stick with your exercise program.

Every time I work out, I think of something small I want to accomplish,

Get Inspired to Get Strong

Need inspiration to work out? Take a look at my average training day in the winter and summer. The next time you think about skipping the gym, think of me: I'm probably either working out, getting ready to work out, or have just finished a workout.

My Average Training Day: Summer

8:00 a.m.
Wake up

8:15 a.m.
Walk Leo and Bear

8:30 a.m.
Breakfast

9:00 a.m.–11:30 a.m.
Strength workout

- 10-minute aerobic warm-up on the bike
- 5 minutes of dynamic stretching
- 5 minutes of muscle activation
- 5 minutes of agility ladder
- 20 minutes of plyometrics
- 60 minutes of weight-lifting exercises
- 10-minute aerobic cooldown on the bike

12 p.m.
Recovery snack

12:30 p.m.–1:15 p.m.
Massage

1:30 p.m.
Lunch

2:00 p.m.–4:00 p.m.
Nap

4:00 p.m.
Snack

4:30 p.m.–6:30 p.m.
Cardio workout

- 90-minute bike ride
- 5 minutes of static stretching

6:30 p.m.
Dinner

7:00 p.m.
Ice knee while watching TV

9 p.m.
Lights out!

My Average Training Day: **Winter**

5:30 a.m.
Wake up

5:45 a.m.–6:30 a.m.
Warm-up for the day
- 15-minute warm-up on the bike, with 8 10-second sprints
- 5 minutes of dynamic stretching
- 2 minutes of agility ladder
- 5 minutes of muscle activation exercises (targeted activities that help ensure you use all your muscles during a workout—read more on page 144)
- 5 minutes of plyometric exercises
- 5 minutes of core exercises

6:30 a.m.
Breakfast

8:15 a.m.–11:00 a.m.
Skiing
- 2 warm-up runs
- Free skiing runs
- 4–6 training runs at high intensity
- Free skiing runs

12:00 p.m.
Lunch

1:00 p.m.–2:00 p.m.
Nap

2:30 p.m.
Snack

3:00 p.m.–4:30 p.m.
Cardio workout
- 45-minute bike ride
- 30 minutes of core exercises
- 20 minutes of balance-improving exercises

4:40 p.m.
Recovery snack

4:45 p.m.–5:45 p.m.
Massage

6:00 p.m.
Dinner

7 p.m.–8 p.m.
Review training or racing videos with coaches

8:30 p.m.
Warm bath with Epsom salts

9 p.m.
Lights out!

whether it's to do more reps, lift a slightly heavier weight, or pump out higher watts on my indoor trainer than the last time I worked out. During my workout, I'll focus on how good hitting my mini-goal will feel instead of how difficult a certain exercise is or how much longer I have to ride the bike. While my mini-goals are usually insignificant, they definitely help me get to the gym and all the way through workouts on a regular basis.

Your mini-goals can be exercise-specific like mine, but they don't have to be. For example, your mini-goal may be to feel slightly more toned in a dress for a big date or to feel better about your body in a bikini when you leave for vacation at the end of the week. In short, whatever you have to tell yourself that helps you get to the gym and through your workout is a great mini-goal to set.

6 **USE ANYTHING AND EVERYTHING TO MAKE YOUR WORKOUT MORE ENJOYABLE.** I know some exercise purists who say you shouldn't read or watch TV when you're working out, because if you can do either, you're not working out hard enough. I don't buy that because I don't think exercise needs to be that exhausting to change your body (see number 4 on page 122), and if watching TV or reading gets you in the gym and helps you continue working out, I'm all for it.

I almost always watch movies or shows when I'm cycling inside. In fact, I can get so immersed in a movie while I'm on the bike that I can forget I'm even exercising!

When I'm not watching TV, I listen to music. Rap, hip-hop, and pop all motivate me to keep going, and I've learned to focus on the one song that's playing at any given time to help me feel good in the moment rather than wondering how much time I have left.

While I don't typically work out with friends, if you find that having a partner motivates you, by all means, do it. The same goes for hiring a trainer. If paying someone or having a personal coach helps get you to the gym on a regular basis, it's money well spent.

7 **SIT LESS.** A big reason many people have a difficult time motivating themselves to exercise is because they spend most of their day doing one thing: sitting. The more you sit, the more likely you are to feel tired and unmotivated to do anything in general—and the less likely you are to want to work out. Most people spend 50 to 70 percent of every day sitting, so it's not surprising that many find it difficult to work out.

How can prolonged sitting sabotage your workout? When we sit for hours on end, studies show that metabolism slows, the electrical activity in our muscles starts to shut down, and our hip flexors and back muscles shorten and weaken. Since our bodies equate prolonged sitting with going to sleep, the more we sit, the more tired we become. Without physical movement to pump blood and oxygen to our brains, our cognitive function also starts to drop, as our brains begin to produce fewer and fewer mood-enhancing chemicals. All this leads to lethargy, physical weakness, and poor mood, making the idea of exercise highly unappealing.

But you don't have to quit your desk job. The good news is that simply standing up more often and taking a few extra walks around your office are enough to counter the effects that prolonged sitting can have on your motivation to work out. Here are simple things you can do to combat sitting's sabotaging effect:

At Work

- Set a timer to chime every twenty minutes, then stand up, walk around your office, and sit back down.

- Take one call per day standing up.

- Walk to a colleague's office instead of emailing.

- Leave your office at least once a day, even if it's just to walk to your car and back.

- Drink more. This has a twofold purpose: You'll stay hydrated, and you'll be forced to get up more frequently to go to the bathroom.

- Ask your HR department for a standing desk or a Swiss ball. Standing desks are becoming more popular options for companies to offer, while sitting on a ball can help strengthen muscles and improve posture.

- Take the stairs, not the elevator.

- Every second counts: Research shows that a two-minute walk every hour is enough to counter the negative effects of sitting.

At Home

- Find a way to make walking part of your daily routine. Most people can't walk to work, but maybe you can walk to the train, bus, or subway. If you drive, consider parking farther away or in another parking lot altogether.

- Walk to shop. If you live in a rural or suburban area, find a complex with several stores that you can walk between, or if you live in a city, walk to a nearby market, even if it means paying slightly more (think of it as an investment in your body).

- Don't drive around to find the closest parking space. Bonus: Your car is less likely to be dented by others when you park farther away from the entrance.

- After dinner, take a five-minute walk outside or even around your home. Doing so will also stimulate blood flow, which improves digestion.

- Enlist your family to be active with you as often as possible. Propose a nightly walk or suggest that each member does one household chore like washing the dishes or taking out the trash during commercial breaks when watching TV.

- Instead of the usual date night of dinner and a movie, see an exhibit at a museum (you'll stand the entire time), go dancing, or go bowling.

- Find ways to stay active while visiting with friends. Propose hiking, skiing, or playing tennis or golf together. Or meet to walk around the local park instead of sitting at the usual coffee shop.

8 RETHINK HOW YOU THINK ABOUT EXERCISE. Growing up in Minnesota, my siblings and I were always playing games, sledding with friends, climbing trees, biking places, clambering on the jungle gym, and in general, being active, rambunctious kids. We never once thought that we were exercising, of course, but all that playing throughout the day definitely amounted to more than one workout.

Many people think the only way to get fit and lean is by going to a gym or running or biking outside for at least twenty minutes at a time. In reality, though, research shows that you can tone muscles and burn just as many (if not more) calories than you do during exercise simply by moving your body more throughout the day. While I still encourage you to find and do a sustained workout that you love at least three days a week, adding more movement to your daily routine will help you get stronger and leaner much faster. Here are some of the ways I love to move my body during the day:

- **Dance around the house** with your favorite song blaring. This is also a great way to blow off steam.

- **Get a cruiser bike.** I love riding my cruiser around town. It may not be raising my heart rate as much as riding a road bike or an indoor Spin bike, but it's still moving my legs and is better than sitting on the couch.

- **Play Wii Fit**, Wii Tennis, Just Dance, or any other active video game.

- **Play a musical instrument.** I can't play any instruments, but I'm jealous of people who can. Studies show that playing the violin for an hour burns as many calories as briskly walking for the same amount of time.

- **Go to a playground** with your kids or relatives' children and go down the slide. Then climb the monkey bars. This will not only get you moving more but will make you feel young and energized.

- **Start a garden.** Gardening is a great way to burn calories. Another bonus: You'll have beautiful flowers for your house or fresh vegetables for your meals.

- **Wash your car.** Do all that hosing and scrubbing, and not only will you burn a ton of calories, you'll also have a cleaner car to show for it.

- **Roughhouse** with your kids, your neighbor's kids, or your dog.

- **Volunteer** at a soup kitchen, for a housing nonprofit, for a Big Brothers Big Sisters organization, or at my own Lindsey Vonn Foundation. In any instance, you'll be standing up to serve food, banging nails to build houses, or playing with kids.

- **Take on a DIY home project** like painting a room or reupholstering a couch.

- **Cook.** Cooking keeps you on your feet—plus, it's the best way to make sure you're eating mostly whole foods.

9 **STAY PRESENT.** I try as hard as possible to stay present in the moment. Whether I'm excited before a big competition, dealing with an injury, or just impatient to get on the hill and get results, I remind myself that all I have is this one moment and that I'd better enjoy it. I focus on the task at hand instead of looking too far down the road or worrying about the future in general.

When I'm training, I try to have the same mind-set and focus on the task at hand and really enjoy what I'm doing in the moment. If I start to get anxious about how much time I have left to work out, I'll double down on paying attention to a movie or listening to the song in my headphones. I'll drape a towel over the clock so I don't obsess over the time, or if I'm lifting weights, I'll focus on executing good form. When I'm cycling outside, I try not to think about an upcoming hill or how far left I have to ride, but let myself get absorbed by my surroundings instead.

But if I have a two-hour ride and I'm already thinking about how much time I have left after fifteen minutes, I'll force myself to stop. Some other athletes and coaches might find that shocking, but I know that I won't get everything I want out of my workout when I'm dreading it that much. So I'll put off the workout for a few hours and try to tackle it again later in the day, when, hopefully, I'm in a different mind-set.

Staying in the moment can also help you push through the physical discomfort that can come with exercise, especially if you haven't worked out in a while. For example, tell yourself that you have to exercise for only one more minute; then when that minute's up, tell yourself to do another minute. Pretty soon you'll find that you've walked twenty minutes without even noticing it.

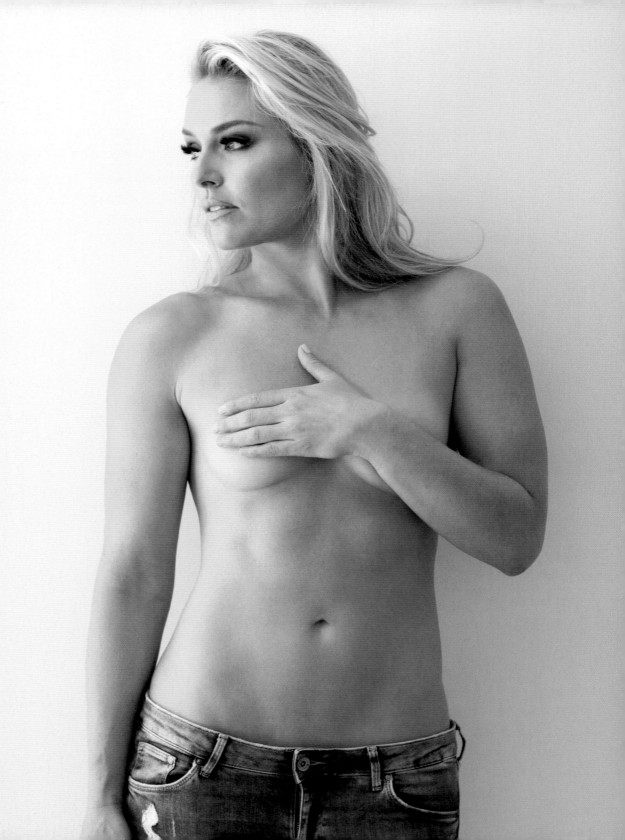

SEVEN AMAZING REASONS TO START STRENGTH TRAINING

One reason I love to strength train is that it makes me feel incredibly empowered. Lifting a heavy weight, pulling a barbell, or balancing on a Swiss ball takes 100 percent of my physical and mental energies, and when I do it right, I feel like a champion, like I've accomplished something small but amazing in a matter of minutes. When I'm in the weight room, I feel focused, purposeful, and powerful, and once I leave, I can feel every muscle fiber quivering in my body, as though I'm instantly tighter, leaner, longer, and stronger—because I am.

Yet I know many women who don't do any strength work because they think it'll make them bulky or won't help them lose weight or they're just intimidated by the idea altogether. But lifting or doing some kind of resistance training is absolutely essential to losing weight, if that's your goal, and a critical part of getting strong, not just physically, but mentally, too. Here are seven ways strength training improves your body and why you need it to get strong and lean.

1 STRENGTH TRAINING IS THE BEST WAY TO DROP FAT AND BUILD MUSCLE. If you want to get super toned—and stay that way—start strength training. Why? Simply put, doing only aerobic exercise won't shape your body as effectively as combining it with resistance work, too. Cardio can't build muscle like lifting weights can; in fact, doing too much aerobic exercise can cause you to lose muscle.

The truth is, you need both strength training and cardio to burn fat and build muscle. Combining the two can cause you to burn up to 40 percent more fat than aerobic exercise alone, which can cause fat *and* muscle loss, studies show. This is partly due to the fact that muscle burns more calories than fat, so the more muscle you have, the more calories your body will use throughout the day. Moreover, the metabolic burn you get after strength training lasts longer because your body needs more energy to repair and rebuild muscle than it does to recover from a cardio workout.

Finally, in case you were wondering: You do burn approximately the same number of calories when you strength train as when you do aerobic exercise if you limit your rest time between exercises. The best way to do this is by combining several resistance moves into one continuous circuit, then rotate through the exercises with minimal rest. To learn how to do this and see nine awesome circuits, flip to chapter 11.

2 NO, YOU WON'T GET BULKY. Worrying that you'll add a ton of muscle by lifting weights is like being afraid that you'll unintentionally get invited to compete at the World Cup because you started skiing every weekend. In other words, your body simply can't and won't manufacture enough testosterone to make you huge—unless you attempt to become a female bodybuilder and start lifting super-heavy weights every day.

But if you're worried about building bulk in the first place, I'd ask yourself why it is that you don't want to have more muscle on your body. Being strong and toned is healthy, feminine, and sexy, and I've never met anyone, male or female, who doesn't agree.

When you start a strength-training program, don't expect your bathroom scale to budge—actually a good sign, as it means you're gaining muscle, which weighs more than fat. Ultimately, the more muscle you have, the easier it will be to burn calories and lose fat. Instead of using the scale, consider measuring your progress by how your clothes fit—a better indicator of changes in body mass. I know from personal experience that you can "gain" a few pounds but actually drop a dress size because you're leaner, tighter, and more toned.

3   **LEARN TO DO BODYWEIGHT WORK, AND THE WORLD BECOMES YOUR GYM.** You don't need to belong to a gym to start strength training. If you can learn a few basic bodyweight exercises, you can get in an incredible workout anywhere—at home, in a hotel room, on the beach, at the playground, or just about anywhere else you can think of. Bodyweight training means using your own bodyweight as resistance to do simple exercises like push-ups, planks, lunges, standing squats, and plyometrics. See chapter 11 for my favorite bodyweight and plyometric exercises, along with ways to combine them into different challenging workouts.

Being able to work out anywhere at any time isn't the only benefit to bodyweight training. Here are some other cool advantages you'll get by learning to do bodyweight work:

- **You'll use more muscles.** Bodyweight exercises recruit more muscles at one time than fixed machines, giving you a better total body workout in less time.

- **You'll burn more calories.** Bodyweight training, especially plyometrics, can require more energy than traditional lifting and even some aerobic exercise.

- **You'll get a stronger core.** When performed properly, bodyweight training is one of the best ways to improve core strength and build muscle tone around your midsection and pelvis.

- **You'll prevent injuries.** Bodyweight training helps strengthen smaller, underutilized muscles that are key to thwarting injuries.

- **You'll get an aerobic and a strength workout at the same time.** By combining bodyweight and plyometric exercises into one circuit, you can get just as much of a heart-pumping aerobic workout as you would doing traditional aerobic exercise. See pages 230 to 231 for my nine favorite circuit workouts.

4 **PREVENT AND TREAT INJURIES—AND POSSIBLY GET RID OF CHRONIC PAIN FOR GOOD—BY STARTING TO STRENGTH TRAIN.** All of us have weak muscles and connective tissue—even I do!—and working to strengthen them can do more to prevent and treat injuries and ailments than almost all other forms of physical exercise. Strength training is effective at ridding chronic injuries and pain because it recruits and conditions smaller muscles that help stabilize and support larger muscles and joints while improving range of motion and helping to correct the muscle imbalances most of us have.

But don't expect relief by going to the gym and haphazardly throwing some weights around; in fact, that's a good way to get injured. Pay close attention to proper form when you lift or do any kind of resistance work. Be sure to follow my instructions closely for the bodyweight and plyometric exercises detailed in chapter 11.

If you're currently injured or suffer from back pain or any other serious physical discomfort, see a doctor before starting a strength-training program.

5 **IMPROVE YOUR HEALTH IN WAYS THAT AEROBIC EXERCISE CAN'T.** Cardio isn't the only gold standard when it comes to improving health through exercise. Resistance training also boosts physical health, even in some ways that aerobic exercise can't.

If you're concerned about bone health, for example, strength training stresses the musculoskeletal system with a weighted load, which in turn prevents bone loss and stimulates new growth. While walking and running also stress bones in the legs, only strength work fortifies bones in your spine and upper body.

Resistance work also increases blood flow to your arms and legs in a different way from aerobic exercise, helping stimulate a longer-lasting drop in blood pressure.

Worried about diabetes or high blood sugar? Like aerobic exercise, strength training improves insulin sensitivity and blood glucose levels while working to help fight hunger and cravings.

Strength training is even good for your brain, with some studies showing that it can be more effective at preventing Alzheimer's and other forms of dementia than aerobic exercise. Some doctors believe that you can even treat cancer with strength training, which has been shown to increase survival rates among those diagnosed with the disease.

6 **START STRENGTH TRAINING, AND YOU'LL BE HAPPIER THAN IF YOU JUST DO AEROBIC EXERCISE.** Just like cardio, strength training boosts mood and emotional well-being by raising levels of endorphins, or hormones that ease pain and stress. But strength training also has unique advantages that you might not necessarily see when doing cardio exercise only.

Studies show that the more muscle you have, the more mood-enhancing chemicals and hormones your body produces over time. That's a pretty great reason in itself to want more muscle, I think! Moreover, strength training is more effective at aligning and improving posture than cardio is, helping increase blood and oxygen flow to the brain and triggering feelings of energy and optimism.

7 **ALLOW YOURSELF TO FEEL MORE BEAUTIFUL.** Want to feel sexy, strong, toned, and beautiful? Start strength training. Research shows that adding resistance work to any regular exercise routine improves body image in women in ways that cardio training may not.

What's so special about strength training? For one, it allows women to accomplish measurable goals, whether lifting more weight, doing more reps, or simply acquiring the skills needed to strength train. Having measurable goals makes progress real and quantifiable—something that psychologists say empowers women more than men.

Studies also show that women feel mentally and emotionally stronger when they lift, regardless of whether they become physically stronger. In one study, women told researchers that after undergoing a strength-training program they felt like they could accomplish things they never thought possible. Part of this has to do with overcoming those old stereotypes that women can't or shouldn't be strong and powerful, which is a liberating and self-satisfying feeling in itself.

Something else happens when women start to strength train, too: They feel better about themselves when they look in the mirror. This is true in my own experience, but it's also a conclusion made by researchers: One study discovered that college-age women who lifted weights for just twelve weeks felt more satisfied with how they looked, even though some gained weight during the study period (the study did not control dorm-room eating). Other research shows that resistance training improves body image better than aerobic exercise. Strength work has even been used to treat women with anorexia because it's been found to be so effective at improving overall body image.

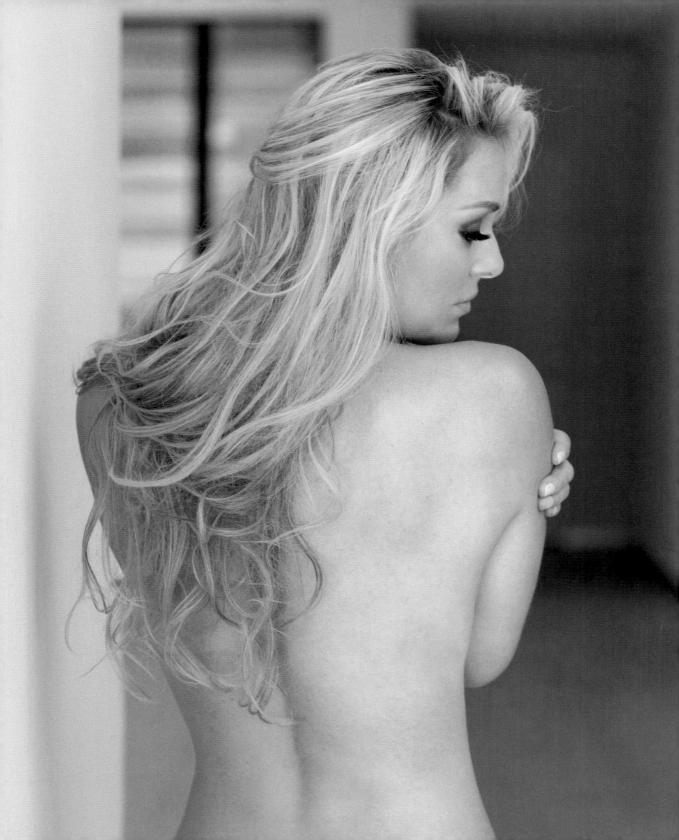

10/ HOW TO WARM UP, STRETCH, AND PREVENT INJURIES

After two major knee surgeries and with one that's only partially functional now, I don't have a choice whether I warm up: It's mandatory. But ever since I started doing so before all my workouts, I can't believe how much the few minutes it takes to warm up have not only strengthened my knee but also helped me overhaul my body to make me fitter, stronger, and leaner than I was before. Yes, I'm talking about getting leaner from a warm-up, not even your workout. What do I do to warm up? I bike, stretch, and perform some basic exercises, all of which are detailed in this chapter and will take you only five to ten minutes total.

I also use the time during my warm-up to create a playlist for the rest of my workout, which psyches me up to go harder and helps me get in the best possible session I can that day.

You already know that I love exercising to music, but the beat has to match my mood if I'm going to really enjoy it and get everything I can out of my workout. Plus, if you always listen to the same music when you exercise, it starts to feel monotonous—and that's about the last thing you want in the gym.

When I'm warming up on the bike, I'll scroll through my phone and choose a set of songs I know will pump me up based on how I feel that day. If I'm frustrated or even angry about something, I'll create a playlist that's heavy on hard-core rap. If I'm in a relaxed mood, I'll choose R&B and pop. Or if I'm really zoned out and having a hard time concentrating, I'll opt for techno-pop. Choosing music to match my mood inspires and motivates me to push harder and get through my workout.

Creating a playlist doesn't just help me work out harder, it also makes me enjoy the physical act of warming up. Warm-ups can feel trivial and like a nuisance at times, but instead of just going through the motions or letting my mind wander to whatever I'm worrying about, I know that I have this cool task to do, playing DJ and making sure that my workout feels like the party it can be.

Why Warming Up Is Key to Getting Strong and Lean

On the rare occasions when I don't warm up before a workout, I usually end the session feeling as if I wasted time in the gym because I wasn't able to bike as hard or lift as much weight. I get angry with myself, swearing that I'll never skip a warm-up again. The next morning I'll often wake up with a sore back or an achy knee—so achy sometimes that I feel like I can't even walk—which helps remind me to stick to my promise.

No matter what kind of workout you're doing, whether a cardio or strength session, a good warm-up (or easing slowly into aerobic exercise) will help ensure that any workout you do is helping make you strong and lean, not wasting your time and energy. Here's how warming up can improve your body and your workout.

DID YOU KNOW?
Being Active Can Burn More Calories Than the Gym

The average woman in the 1950s burned nearly double the number of calories the average woman does today. More incredibly, the 1950s female wasn't burning all these calories on a treadmill or in a Flywheel class. Instead, women did more physical housework, walked their children to and from school, walked to shops, and were busy preparing and cooking dinner. While I'm not suggesting that you adopt the regimen of a 1950s housewife, it goes to show how simply making more nonexercise activity part of your daily routine can help you start to get strong, with or without the gym.

The Four Best Ways to Warm Up

1 **AEROBIC EXERCISE.** It may seem silly to exercise before you exercise, but that's exactly what you have to do if you want to get the most out of any workout. Warming up with some light cardio like spinning or walking raises your internal temperature and increases oxygen and blood flow to your muscles and brain, helping prepare you physically and mentally for exercise. If you're doing an aerobic workout like jogging, biking, or using a cardio machine at the gym, simply start at a slower pace or a lower resistance before going into full workout mode. If you're strength training, spend a few minutes walking or biking first to get warm and loose.

2 **MUSCLE ACTIVATION.** If you've never heard of muscle activation, you're not alone: Most people aren't familiar with the technique. But once you learn how much it can help tone your body and rev your workout, I guarantee you'll be telling all your friends.

Muscle activation exercises recruit your body's weakest or most underused muscles, literally activating them or turning them on so that you can use them during exercise. For most people, the most underused muscles are the glutes and the core. Activating these muscle groups before a workout ensures that they get used, not allowed to grow weaker and weaker. This means you also get a full-body workout, which will boost your total caloric burn. My favorite muscle activation exercises are walking lunges, planks (page 210), glute bridges (page 216), and lateral resistance band walks (page 229).

3 **DYNAMIC STRETCHING.** Gone are the days when top-level athletes did a ton of static stretching—what you did as a kid in gym class

Ten Ways Warming Up Can Transform Your Workout

1. Helps you exercise harder and longer so you can get fitter and leaner

2. Triggers hormones that help burn fat before you even start working out

3. Makes exercise more comfortable by helping your muscles relax more quickly

4. Prevents overheating by stimulating the sweat process earlier

5. Lessens the stress on your heart and other organs during your workout

6. Increases the range of motion in your spine, knees, hips, and other joints

7. Gives you time to prepare mentally for your workout so you can give it your all

8. Helps your muscles recover faster after you stop working out

9. Significantly lowers the chances that you'll get injured

10. Significantly lowers the chances that you'll feel sore or achy the next day

when you had to touch your toes. Holding stretches in the same position for a period of time has been shown to increase inflammation and possibly cause injuries rather than prevent them. Instead, most elite athletes now do dynamic stretching, or exercises that move their muscles through a controlled pattern. Similar to muscle activation, dynamic stretching helps recruit weak or underused muscles while increasing blood flow and oxygen to the limbs and honing balance and coordination.

Dynamic stretching also prepares your muscles and joints in a unique way for exercise by taking your body through motions similar to those you'll do when you work out. For example, front leg swings, a

Lindsey's Playlists

When I'm Frustrated or Need an Extra Push

1. "Touch'N You," Rick Ross ft. Usher
2. "She Will," Lil Wayne ft. Drake
3. "Trillionaire," Bun B ft. T-Pain
4. "Motivation," Kelly Rowland ft. Lil Wayne
5. "Red Nation," The Game ft. Lil Wayne
6. "Headlines," Drake
7. "Starships," Nicki Minaj
8. "No Lie," 2 Chainz ft. Drake
9. "Toot It and Boot It," Slugga Black ft. YG
10. "Self Made," DJ Drama ft. Red Cafe & Yo Gotti

When I'm in a Good Mood but Need to Focus

1. "If It Ain't Love," Jason Derulo
2. "YOUTH," Troye Sivan
3. "Working For It," ZHU, Skrillex & THEY.
4. "Fast Car," Jonas Blue ft. Dakota
5. "Lush Life," Zara Larsson
6. "Sit Still, Look Pretty," Daya
7. "Say My Name (Hermitude Remix)," ODESZA ft. Zyra
8. "Confident," Demi Lovato
9. "On Purpose," Dougie F ft. Pitbull
10. "The Buzz," Hermitude ft. Big K.R.I.T., Mataya & Young Tapz

When I'm Feeling Relaxed

1. "Sweet Love," Chris Brown
2. "Can't Be Friends," Trey Songz
3. "Let Me Love You," Mario
4. "Ice Box," Omarion
5. "In Those Jeans," Ginuwine
6. "Pot of Gold," The Game ft. Chris Brown
7. "Long Way 2 Go," Cassie
8. "Ride," Ciara ft. Ludacris
9. "Got 'Til It's Gone," Janet Jackson ft. Q-Tip and Joni Mitchell
10. "Turn Your Lights Down Low," Bob Marley and the Wailers

When I'm Getting Ready to Race

1. "Champion," Chipmunk ft. Chris Brown
2. "Say What You Want," Future ft. Pastor AD3
3. "Who Gon Stop Me," Kanye West ft. Jay-Z
4. "Beez in the Trap," Nicki Minaj ft. 2 Chainz
5. "Imma Do It," Fabolous ft. Kobe
6. "Remember the Name," Fort Minor ft. Styles of Beyond
7. "She Will," Lil Wayne ft. Drake
8. "Steady Mobbin," Young Money ft. Gucci Mane
9. "Heroes (We Could Be)," Alesso
10. "Do It Like a Dude," Jessie J

common dynamic stretch, will help get your body ready to move your legs when you run or use an elliptical, reducing the risk of injury while boosting your performance.

My favorite dynamic stretches are walking quad stretches (page 228) and walking hamstring stretches; both help loosen my hips and quads, which are perpetually tight. Other dynamic stretches include walking knee hugs, side leg swings, walking leg swings, and catch and release quad stretches.

The Ultimate Twelve-Minute Warm-Up

- **Two minutes of foam roller work.** If you have tight muscles to loosen, spend two minutes on a foam roller before you stretch and do activation.

- **Five minutes of light aerobic exercise.** Start by walking briskly, biking or spinning at a low resistance, or using a cardio machine at a reduced pace or low resistance.

- **Five minutes of dynamic stretching and muscle activation.** Spend the last five minutes doing a muscle activation exercise and several dynamic stretches that target the muscles that you'll use during your workout. (See pages 228 and 229 for examples.)

4 FOAM ROLLING. Most people are familiar with foam rollers or those cylindrical tubes you can use to roll and relieve tightness in your IT band, back, glutes, hamstrings, and other trigger points. While foam rollers are most often used for massage or for recovery from injuries, they can also help warm up muscles and connective tissue when used before a workout. Using a foam roller before exercise specifically breaks down adhesions, or sticky points, between fascia (sheets of connective tissue) and muscles. This helps increase muscles' elasticity and extensibility, limiting tightness during workouts to improve performance and prevent injuries.

Foam rolling—or any type of self-massage—also has a unique secondary benefit: It releases chemicals in your brain that stimulate relaxation and block feelings of fatigue, helping you push harder during workouts.

Five Steps to Prevent and Deal with Injuries

Starting to warm up on a regular basis will help you prevent injuries and relieve aches and pains. But a good warm-up alone isn't enough to totally thwart the risk of injuries. As I've learned the hard way, you need a few more tricks up your sleeve if you want to get strong and lean (and stay that way) without watching your hard work suddenly evaporate because of some silly mistake.

The good news: Warming up may be the most time-consuming step you need to take to prevent injuries. My other recommendations that follow are more about attitude shift and follow-through if you do happen to get injured. Just remember: Being in pain or injured is no fun, trust me. No matter your goals or what you do for a workout, it's absolutely essential to do everything you can to make sure that you can move—and continue to move—with all the grace, elegance, and efficiency that you possess. Here are my top five steps to keep your body moving and continuing to look strong and lean.

1 LISTEN TO YOUR BODY. This sounds easy enough, but few people actually pay attention to how they feel. But if you don't take the time to listen to your body, you can easily undo whatever hours you spend in the gym or all that eating healthy in a matter of a few minutes during one workout.

I'm an elite athlete, but it's taken me years to learn to listen to my body, and it's something I still struggle with today. It's part of my personality to push, push, push, with my foot pressed down on the pedal all the time. Yet as I've learned through trial and error, driving full speed toward your goals without easing up now and then to check in with how you feel can quickly prevent yourself from reaching your goals.

But how exactly do you listen to your body? Here are three ways to start.

- **Keep a workout journal or use wearables.** Whether you invest in a wearable technology that tracks your workouts for you, or you do it the old-fashioned way with a training log, reviewing your exercise efforts and how you feel will force you to check in with your body and pay closer attention to the physical you. Over time, a wearable device or training log can also help you identify useful trends such as whether you feel better exercising in the morning, which foods fuel you the best, and how many strenuous days per week your body can tolerate.

- **Do a bedtime body check.** When you're lying in bed at night, assess how every part of your body feels, starting with your head and neck, then moving through your shoulders, arms, spine, trunk, and hips, ending with the muscles in your legs and feet. Does anything hurt or feel unusually sore? Do some parts of your body feel overtaxed while others feel underworked? How tired are you? If you're too exhausted to do a bedtime check, you probably need to reevaluate your routine (or lack thereof, as being inactive can also make you tired).

- **Get regular massages.** Most people aren't familiar with human anatomy, but getting a regular massage can be as good as getting a crash course in physiology. During a massage, a good masseuse will call attention with her hands to all those muscles, tendons, and ligaments that you might not know even existed. Plus, when someone is digging into any area of your body, you can tell right away if something's unusually sore, tender, or achy.

2 **DON'T PUSH YOURSELF.** Exercise shouldn't be painful—ever. If you haven't worked out in a long time or are doing something challenging or new, you'll likely feel some level of discomfort, and that's totally normal. You'll probably also be sore the next day or two, which is a good thing, as it means your muscles are adapting and getting stronger.

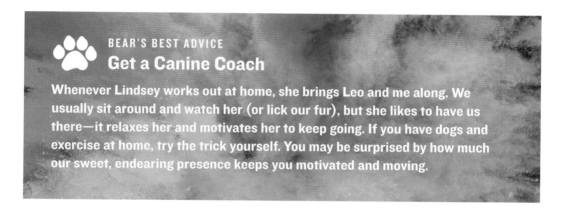

BEAR'S BEST ADVICE
Get a Canine Coach

Whenever Lindsey works out at home, she brings Leo and me along. We usually sit around and watch her (or lick our fur), but she likes to have us there—it relaxes her and motivates her to keep going. If you have dogs and exercise at home, try the trick yourself. You may be surprised by how much our sweet, endearing presence keeps you motivated and moving.

But there's a big difference between being sore and being in pain, and it's important to be able to differentiate between the two. In most instances, pain is sharp and intense. If my knee hurts during a work-out, I know it immediately—it feels like someone is sticking a little knife into the joint. But if my knee is sore, it feels like a dull ache, which doesn't necessarily mean I need to stop working out.

Pain can also limit your mobility or range of motion in a way that soreness can't. I'm not talking about those days when you feel like you can't jump out of bed because you biked up a killer hill or did some new strength routine. But if you start favoring one leg over the other or are consistently unable to reach with one arm for an item on a high shelf, you're likely suffering from a pain that needs to be addressed.

In either case, whether you have pain during or after a workout, don't push through it. If you do, you'll likely end up injured. Similarly, you shouldn't push yourself when you're sick, stressed, or sleep deprived—all which can make your body more susceptible to injury. While exercise can be a great stress reliever and it's typically okay to work out if you just have a head cold (or other illness above the neck), remember to take it easy. When your body is compromised by sickness, stress, or lack of sleep, you should not shoot for all-time record results in the gym.

3 **WARM UP. SERIOUSLY.** Reread the first part of this chapter. Then, no excuses: Take an extra five to ten minutes (shorter than you probably spend waiting in line for coffee) and do it. Warming up is the best way to prevent injuries, plus you'll be boosting your performance and helping your body in a zillion other ways (see page 145 for the top ten ways warming up helps your body get strong).

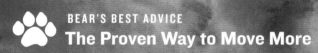

BEAR'S BEST ADVICE
The Proven Way to Move More

If you really want to move more, get a dog (bonus points if you adopt a rescue dog like me). Studies show that 60 percent of all dog owners meet the national criteria for regular exercise, while almost half are active for thirty minutes or more per day at least five times a week. Lindsey's always taking Leo and me for walks, to the park, or out in the backyard to chase marmots. This means I'm helping her be happy as well as stay fit and lean.

4 **COOL DOWN.** I cool down for five to ten minutes after my workouts, usually by doing a quick spin on the bike. While cooling down isn't as beneficial for injury prevention as warming up, it does help flush lactic acid buildup from tired legs and, if you have an injury, can help you stay loose and flexible. Some studies show that cooling down also prevents excess blood from pooling in the muscles—the reason you can feel dizzy or even nauseous if you hop off the bike or treadmill without a recovery period.

For me, there's also a big psychological benefit to cooling down. After I've finished a hard workout and nailed my goal for the day, nothing feels better than taking the time to shake it out while reflecting on what I've accomplished.

5 **DO YOUR PHYSICAL THERAPY—EACH AND EVERY EXERCISE.** If you do happen to get injured, don't wait until you're really in pain or can't move before seeing a medical expert. Make an appointment with a sports medicine doctor or even your family physician as soon as possible. Then once you have a diagnosis, ask your doctor (or get a referral to see a physical therapist) to create a program of strengthening exercises that will help treat the injury and prevent you from getting injured again.

Whatever you do, don't blow off the idea of physical therapy. If you get injured, it means some part of your body is weak—either the injured tissue itself or the area surrounding it. While rest is often necessary to heal, if you remain inactive without strengthening the injury or area around it, it'll just get weaker and weaker, making it more vulnerable to reinjury when you are active again.

After you have a physical therapy program in place, think of it like a prescription: You need to take it every day, as recommended, to get better. Just as with working out, you have to be diligent, putting the same

The Most Luxurious Way to Get Lean

Need more motivation to work out? Tell yourself that you'll get a massage if you meet your weekly or monthly fitness goals. When you want to call it quits, just imagine those hands kneading out your tired muscles.

Massages aren't just great motivation material—they can also prevent injuries, help improve exercise performance, and increase feelings of self-worth.

I've made massage a priority in my weekly schedule for years, and not only because that's what pro athletes do. Massage makes me feel relaxed, rejuvenated, and revitalized, better about myself, my body, and life in general. I believe our bodies are the most valuable thing we own, and your body has to last you longer than any other costly possession like a car or home. So why wouldn't you take the time and effort to pamper and protect it as you would your car or home?

I get massages at least five days a week, even in the off-season. But for most people, just one monthly massage can offer big benefits to your motivation levels, physical performance, and self-esteem.

The best part: You don't have to spend a ton of money to get a good massage. While you should always see a licensed masseuse or physical therapist if you have a specific injury or ailment, if you're just looking to pamper tired muscles, there are a dozen ways to get a great inexpensive massage. When I lived in L.A., for example, I found a fabulous Thai massage place where a good, deep session cost less than takeout. If you live in a big city, try looking for shiatsu, a Japanese form of deep massage; you can often find it at smaller clinics or spas for a reasonable price. Some neighborhood nail salons also offer a short session of deep massage with a manicure or pedicure, which isn't a bad way to spend an afternoon after a hard morning workout.

Many massage schools and university sports clinics offer discounted massages from students in training. Call ahead to ask about special pricing before you book. Some massage chains also give special introductory rates for first-time clients or deep discounts when you commit to buying a number of sessions. And there's nothing wrong with trying a quick chair masseuse if you see someone advertising a good rate. No matter where you get your massage, be sure to drink plenty of water afterward to help your body flush out toxins released during deep tissue work.

amount of time and effort into healing your body as you would into making it strong. That means doing each and every rehab exercise, no matter how insignificant it may seem. It might take extra motivation to get yourself moving when you're still in recovery mode, but trust me, the work will be worth it. All of the time and energy you spend on physical therapy will pay off as your body regains its strength.

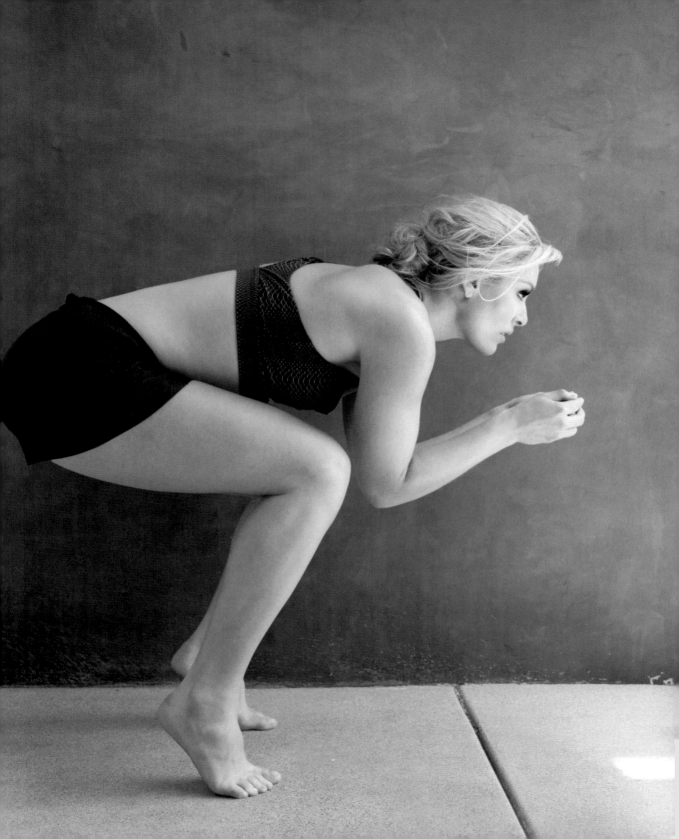

11/
MY 65 FAVORITE GET-STRONG EXERCISES

n this chapter, you'll find the strength-training exercises that I've used to get strong and lean, along with nine circuits that combine the exercises into thirty-minute workouts. You can do these exercises and circuits at any time and anywhere—in your living room, at the gym, in your backyard, in a hotel room. You don't already have to have a certain amount of muscle, specific body type, or any experience to do them, either. Simply follow these steps to start overhauling your health and transforming your body today.

1 FIND YOUR FITNESS LEVEL.

● **Beginner**: You're a beginner if you haven't worked out in several months (or years) or simply don't feel comfortable with strength training.

■ **Intermediate**: You're an intermediate if you have experience with strength training and have a base level of muscle strength and cardiovascular fitness.

◆ **Expert**: You're an expert if you have experience with strength training, have been working out regularly for more than one year, and have a solid level of muscle strength and cardiovascular fitness.

2 GET FAMILIAR WITH THE EXERCISES.
If you've been to a gym, ever picked up a fitness magazine, or watched a workout DVD, many of my exercises will look familiar, even if you've never tried them yourself. But before you start, take a minute to familiarize yourself by looking at the picture and reading the description. For each exercise in your fitness level, tell yourself, *I can do that*—because you can.

The exercises are divided up into five different categories:

- **Power.** These are plyometric exercises that will improve your explosiveness, balance, coordination, and overall fitness while toning your abs, butt, thighs, and calves.

- **Lower-Body Push.** These primarily work the quadriceps and tone your butt, your thighs, and the front of your legs.

- **Upper-Body Push.** These involve pushing and tone your chest, arms, shoulders, and triceps.

- **Lower-Body Pull.** These primarily work your hamstrings and tone your butt, your thighs, and the back of your legs.

- **Upper-Body Pull.** These involve pulling and tone your back and biceps.

- **Core.** These are trunk exercises that will strengthen your hips and pelvis and tone your midsection, abs, butt, and thighs.

If you're doing a circuit, perform the exercises in the order listed above, starting with Power and ending with Core. Power exercises, which involve jumping, raise your heart rate significantly, helping you start a workout on an aerobic level. They are also easier to do when your muscles are fresh, since they're usually the most exhausting. After the muscles in your legs are activated, transition to Lower-Body Push to tone the front of your legs. Before working the back of your legs, give your lower body a break by doing Upper-Body Push exercises. Then, rotate back to Lower-Body Pull to work the back of your legs before transitioning to Upper-Body Pull and Core.

3 GET FAMILIAR WITH THE ACCESSORIES. Most exercises don't require any equipment, but for some, you'll need a set of dumbbells. Unless you plan to train at a gym, invest in a set of 5-pound weights or, better still, several pairs of dumbbells ranging from 5 to 15 pounds. Dumbbell sets aren't expensive; in fact, you can find them for less than what you'd spend eating one dinner out.

FIVE SECONDS TO A STRONGER YOU

How to Use Any Machine at Any Gym

Many machines can look confusing or intimidating at first. Even I don't know how to use some weight-lifting equipment, and I've been strength training for years. But just because you don't know how to use a machine doesn't mean you should avoid it. I simply look at the how-to illustrations posted on the machine. Every single piece of equipment is required to have them, and while it sounds obvious, you can learn almost everything you need to know about proper form by looking at these pictures.

I also recommend investing in a Swiss ball, which will cost you the equivalent of about two movie tickets. (Swiss balls come in various diameters to suit people of different heights, so double-check to be sure you're getting one that is the right size for you.) Having a Swiss ball will help you do a wider variety of bodyweight exercises. It also has the double bonus of serving as a chair when you're watching TV or working from home, helping strengthen and stabilize your core muscles as you sit.

In some exercises, I use a bench at a gym, but if you're at home, you can easily use a chair. Similarly, I use a medicine ball for a few exercises, but at home, you can use a dumbbell and get the same results.

To do my favorite muscle activation exercises, or the lateral resistance band walk, you'll need a resistance band. Most gyms have these, but if you're working out at home, you can find one online or pick one up at a physical therapy or sports medicine clinic, which often sell them for as little as $5.

Finally, some intermediate and expert exercises use a half stability ball, or Bosu ball. If you don't have one and don't want to invest in one, you can also use a balance board or even a pillow.

4 **CHOOSE ONE OF MY CIRCUITS OR CREATE YOUR OWN.** On pages 230 to 231, you'll find nine of my favorite circuit workouts—three for each fitness level with seven exercises each. For each circuit, perform one set of repetitions for the first exercise, then move on to the next exercise listed, taking as little rest as possible between sets, until you've completed one set for all seven exercises. Repeat the circuit three times total. A short recovery time keeps your heart rate elevated, allowing you to get in a cardio and strength workout at the same.

DID YOU KNOW?
Lift to Live Longer

The more muscle mass you have, the less likely you are to die early from any cause, according to research.

You can also create your own circuit by choosing any five to seven exercises and combining them into one routine. For best results, pick exercises that work different muscle groups—for example, one Power, one Lower-Body Push, one Upper-Body Push, one Lower-Body Pull, one Upper-Body Pull, and two Core. If you choose to do only five exercises, omit one Lower-Body, one Upper-Body, and/or one Core exercise.

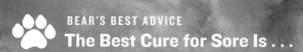

BEAR'S BEST ADVICE
The Best Cure for Sore Is . . .

If I fall into a stream chasing a big stick and my undercarriage gets sore, I know one of the worst things I can do is stop chasing sticks. It may seem counterintuitive to you humans, but sore muscles only get sorer if you don't keep moving. Muscles need blood and oxygen to recover properly, and the best way to get both to them is by staying active! If you're really sore, you don't have to work out, but try to take a walk or a light yoga class. Better yet, if you have dogs, take us on a walk!

5 **WARM UP.** This is critical before strength training. See chapter 10 for more details, but spend at least five minutes doing some light aerobic exercise like walking or spinning, followed by dynamic stretching and muscle activation, before you start any strength work.

6 **STRENGTH TRAIN TWICE A WEEK.** While your body will benefit from any amount of strength training, completing at least two twenty-minute workouts per week will stress your muscles enough to cause visible changes, as well as all those great invisible changes detailed in chapter 9.

Love strength training so much that you want to do it every day? Don't. Your muscles and connective tissue need time to recover in order to adapt. Strength training more than four times a week will cause your body to break down, not grow stronger. On the days you don't strength train, get in some form of cardio—remember, combining the two is the fastest and most effective way to get strong, lean, and healthy while preventing injuries and burnout.

7 **EXPERIMENT!** Just because you're a beginner doesn't mean you can't mix some intermediate exercises into your routine, especially as your strength and comfort improve. Start slowly by incorporating a few intermediate exercises into your circuit, or if you're already an intermediate, try expert exercises that seem suitable to your skill and fitness.

8 **NEVER DO ANYTHING THAT MAKES YOU UNCOMFORTABLE.** You can usually tell if an exercise is feasible for you by looking at the picture and reading the instructions. But if the thought of doing it makes you uncomfortable, even if it's a beginner exercise, don't try it. There's absolutely nothing wrong with waiting until your skill or fitness progresses to experiment. I'm in the weight room almost every day, and there are some exercises that even I won't try.

65 GET-STRONG EXERCISES

POWER

1 | ● ■ ◆ | SPLIT HOPS

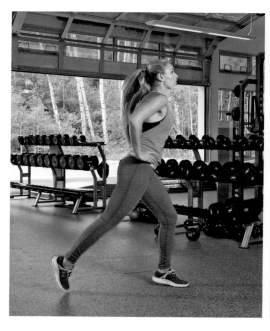 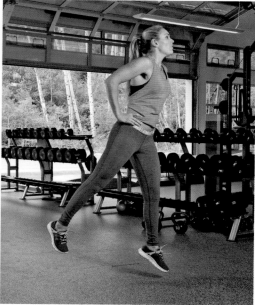

1. Stand with your feet together, toes forward, hands on your hips.

2. Step your right foot back into a split stance, keeping your left foot flat on the floor, right knee slightly bent.

3. With your chest high and head straight, jump as high as possible, switching legs midair to land with your right foot forward, left foot back in a split stance.

4. Jump continuously, scissoring your legs on every jump, until you've completed 12–15 jumps with each leg landing forward (24–30 jumps total).

5. Rest and repeat for 3 sets total.

POWER

1 | ● ■ ◆ | SPLIT SQUAT JUMPS

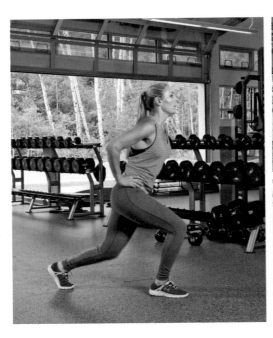 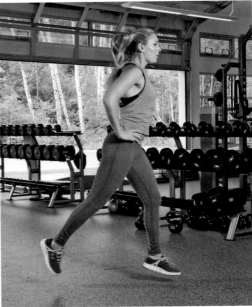

I. Stand with your feet together, toes forward, hands on your hips.

2. Step your left foot back into a split stance, spiking your left heel. With your chest high and head straight, sink into a deep squat, bending both knees as low as possible, then jump as high as possible.

3. Land in the same position, bending your knees on impact to absorb the landing. Straighten your legs to return to the start position.

4. Jump continuously until you've completed 10–12 jumps on that leg. Then switch legs and complete 10–12 jumps on your right leg.

5. Rest and repeat for 3 sets total.

POWER

1 | ●■◆ | SCISSOR JUMPS

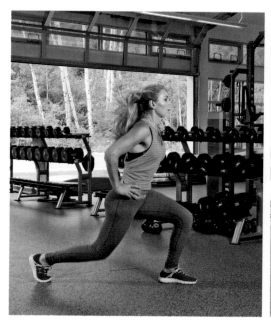 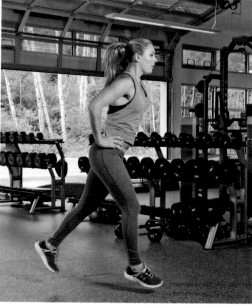

1. Perform the exercise described in the intermediate version, but switch your feet midair while jumping so that you land with a different foot forward on every jump.

2. Complete 8–10 jumps with each leg landing forward (16–20 jumps total).

3. Rest and repeat for 3 sets total.

POWER

2 | ●■◆ | SQUAT JUMPS

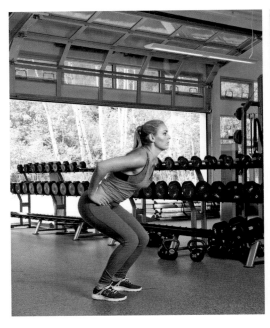 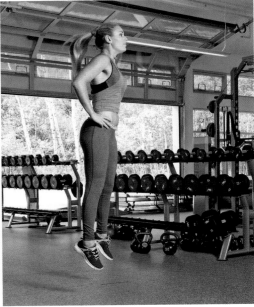

1. Stand with your feet shoulder-width apart, toes forward, hands on your hips.

2. Sink into a deep squat by sitting your butt down and back, keeping your back flat and your weight on your heels.

3. Jump as high as possible, keeping hands on your hips and head straight.

4. Land, bending your knees on impact, then straighten your legs to return to the start position.

5. Jump continuously until you've completed 12–15 jumps.

6. Rest and repeat for 3 sets total.

POWER

2 | ● ■ ◆ | TUCK JUMPS

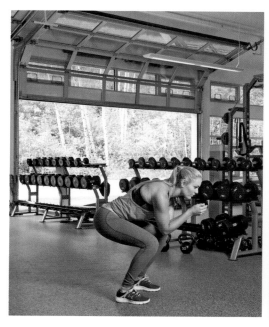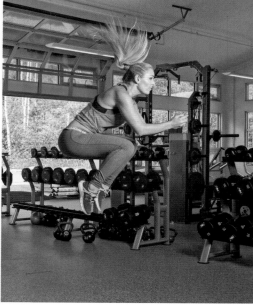

1. Stand with your feet hip-width apart, toes forward, knees slightly bent, elbows bent, hands clasped in front of you.

2. Jump as high as possible, lifting both knees to your chin without bending your upper body forward.

3. Land, bending your knees on impact, then immediately jump again, bringing knees to chin.

4. Jump continuously until you've completed 10–12 jumps.

5. Rest and repeat for 3 sets total.

POWER

2 | ●■◆ | SQUAT JUMPS WITH A DUMBBELL

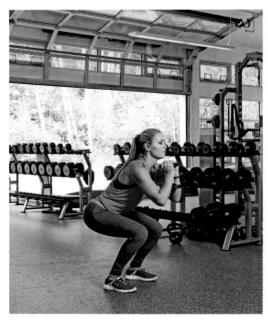 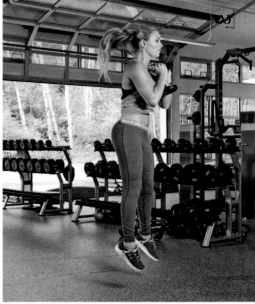

1. Stand with your feet shoulder-width apart, toes forward. Hold a dumbbell by placing both hands under one handle or end of the weight and pulling it tight to your chest, elbows down, so the weight is parallel with your body.

2. Sink into a deep squat by sitting your butt down and back, keeping your back flat and your weight on your heels.

3. Jump as high as possible, keeping the dumbbell close to your chest and your head straight.

4. Land, bending your knees on impact, then straighten your legs to return to the start position.

5. Jump continuously until you've completed 8–10 jumps.

6. Rest and repeat for 3 sets total.

POWER

3 | ●■◆ | LATERAL LINE HOPS

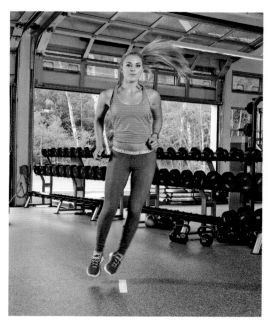 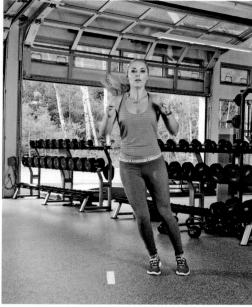

1. Stand with your feet together, toes forward, arms by your side.

2. Jump sideways to the right with both feet, keeping your ankles together and legs straight. Then immediately jump sideways to the left, as if jumping over an imaginary line under you.

3. Jump continuously, minimizing your contact with the floor, keeping your toes up and ankles stiff.

4. Complete 12–15 jumps to each side.

5. Rest and repeat for 3 sets.

POWER

3 | ●■◆ | LATERAL SKATER HOPS

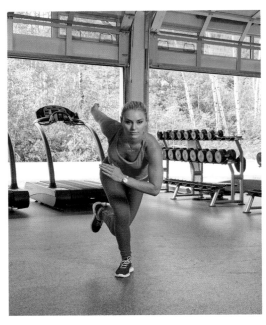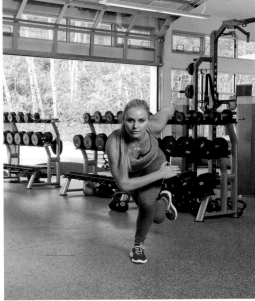

I. Standing in a comfortable stance, hop sideways off your left foot and onto your right foot, absorbing the landing on your right leg by bending the hip, knee, and ankle.

2. Without letting your left foot touch the ground, immediately hop off your right foot and onto your left, absorbing the landing without letting your right foot touch the ground.

3. Repeat in this fashion, jumping back and forth laterally for 10–12 hops to each side.

4. Rest and repeat for 3 sets.

POWER

3 | ●■◆ | LATERAL SKATER BOUNDS

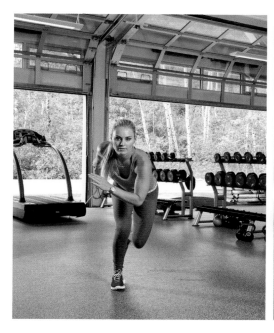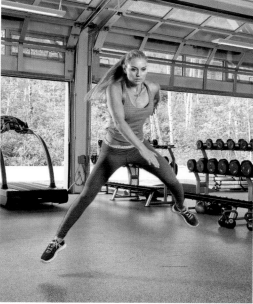

1. Standing in a comfortable stance, jump as far as possible sideways off your left foot and onto your right foot, absorbing the landing on your right leg by bending the hip, knee, and ankle.

2. Without letting your left foot touch the ground, immediately bound off your right foot as far as possible and onto your left, absorbing the landing without letting your right foot touch the ground.

3. Repeat in this fashion, bounding back and forth laterally for 8–10 bounds to each side.

4. Rest and repeat for 3 sets.

LOWER-BODY PUSH

4 | ●■◆ | SIDE SQUATS

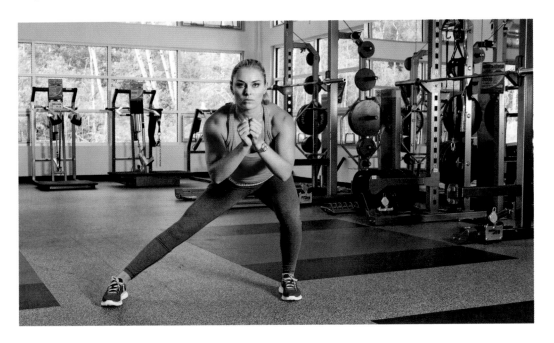

1. Stand with your feet wider than shoulder-width apart, toes forward, hands clasped in front of you.

2. Bend your left knee to sit your weight down and back onto your left leg, keeping your right leg straight, chest high, and shoulder blades down and back.

3. Straighten your left leg to return to the start position.

4. Perform the same movement to the right, alternating legs until you've completed 12–15 squats to each side.

5. Rest and repeat for 3 sets total.

LOWER-BODY PUSH

4 | ●■◆ | SIDE LUNGES WITH A DUMBBELL

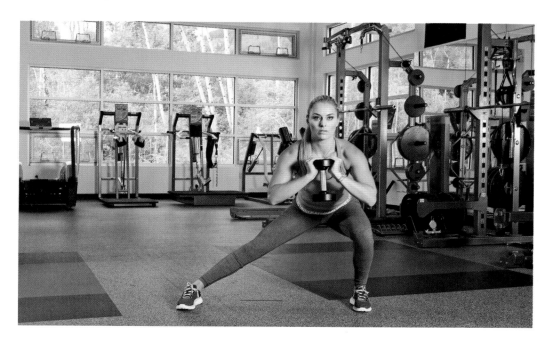

1. Stand with your feet together, toes forward. Hold a dumbbell by placing both hands under the top handle or one end, pulling it to your chest, elbows down, so the weight is parallel with your body.

2. Take a wide step sideways with your left foot, keeping toes forward. Bend your left knee as low as possible to sit your weight down and back onto your left leg, keeping your right leg straight, chest high, and dumbbell close to your chest.

3. Straighten your left leg to return to the start position.

4. Perform the same movement to the right, alternating legs until you've completed 10-12 lunges to either side.

5. Rest and repeat for 3 sets total.

LOWER-BODY PUSH

4 ●■◆ | SIDE LUNGES WITH DUMBBELLS

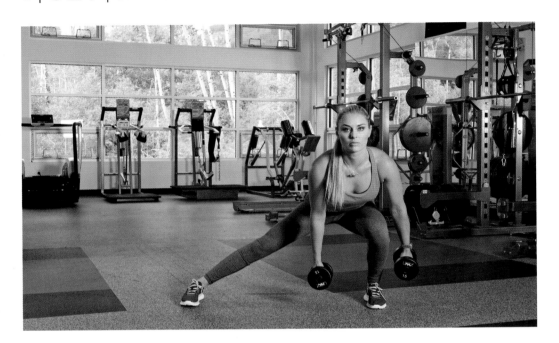

1. Stand with your feet together, toes forward. Hold a dumbbell in each hand, arms by your side.

2. Perform the exercise as described in the intermediate version while letting the dumbbells hang toward the floor on each side lunge.

3. Complete 8–10 lunges to either side.

4. Rest and repeat for 3 sets total.

LOWER-BODY PUSH

5 | ●■◆ | SPLIT SQUATS

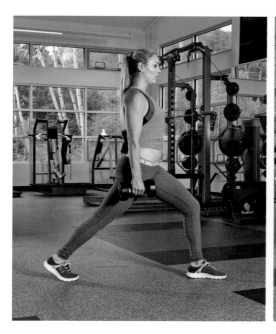 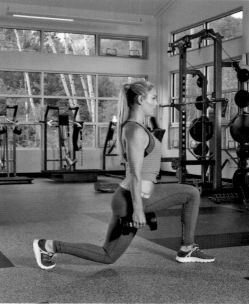

1. Stand on your left leg, toes forward, with a dumbbell in each hand, arms at your sides. Step your right foot back into a split stance, spiking your heel up.

2. With your back flat and eyes forward, sink straight down into a deep squat, bending your knees until your left thigh is parallel with the floor.

3. Slowly straighten to the start position.

4. Complete 12–15 squats on your left leg, then 12–15 squats on your right.

5. Rest and repeat for 3 sets total.

LOWER-BODY PUSH

5 | ● ■ ◆ | REAR-FOOT ELEVATED SPLIT SQUATS WITH DUMBBELLS

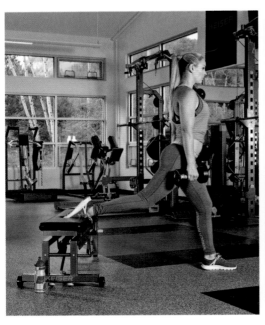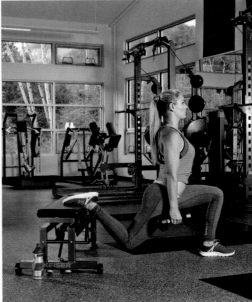

1. Stand balanced, toes forward, placing your right foot and ankle on a step behind you. Hold a dumbbell in each hand, arms by your sides.

2. With your eyes forward, sink straight down into a deep squat, bending your knees until your left thigh is parallel with the step and your right knee touches the floor if possible.

3. Straighten your legs to the start position.

4. Complete 10–12 squats on your left leg, then 10–12 squats on your right.

5. Rest and repeat for 3 sets total.

LOWER-BODY PUSH

5 | ● ■ ◆ | SWISS BALL REAR-FOOT ELEVATED SPLIT SQUATS WITH DUMBBELLS

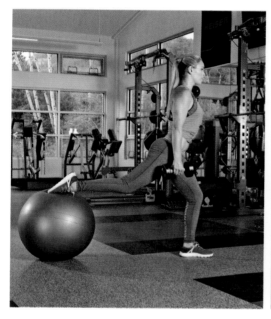 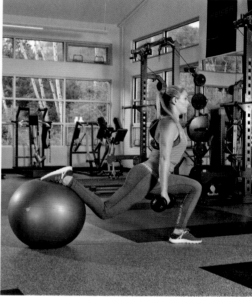

1. Stand balanced, toes forward, with your right foot and ankle on a Swiss ball behind you. Hold a dumbbell in each hand, arms by your sides.

2. With your eyes forward, sink straight down into a deep squat, bending both knees until your left thigh is parallel with the floor, allowing the dumbbells to hang toward the floor.

3. Straighten your legs back to the start position.

4. Complete 8–10 squats on your left leg, then 8–10 squats on your right.

5. Rest and repeat for 3 sets total.

LOWER-BODY PUSH

6 ●■◆ | SQUATS WITH A DUMBBELL

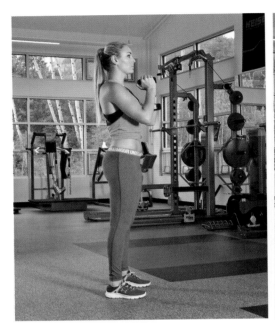 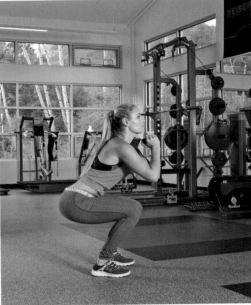

1. Stand with your feet shoulder-width apart, toes forward. Hold a dumbbell by placing both hands under the top handle or end, pulling it to your chest, elbows down, so the weight is parallel with your body.

2. With your eyes forward, sit your butt down and back until your thighs are parallel with the floor, keeping your chest high and your weight on your heels.

3. Straighten your legs back to the start position.

4. Complete 12–15 squats.

5. Rest and repeat for 3 sets total.

LOWER-BODY PUSH

6 ● ■ ◆ | SQUATS WITH DUMBBELLS

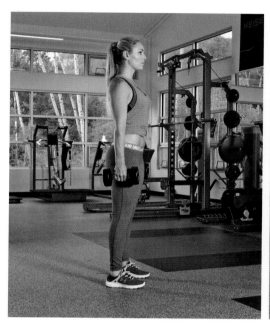 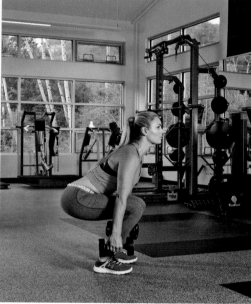

1. Stand with your feet shoulder-width apart, toes forward, with a dumbbell in each hand, arms by your sides.

2. With your eyes forward, sit your butt down and back until your thighs are parallel with the floor, keeping your chest high and your weight on your heels.

3. Straighten your legs back to the start position.

4. Complete 10–12 squats.

5. Rest and repeat for 3 sets total.

LOWER-BODY PUSH

6 | ●■◆ | BARBELL BACK SQUATS

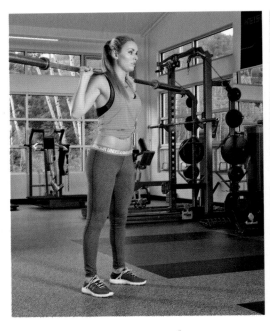 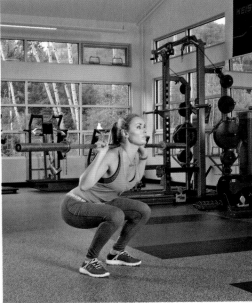

1. Set up a barbell in a squat rack so that the barbell is at the height of your sternum. While the barbell is in the rack, walk under the barbell so that it rests on your shoulders. Squat the barbell out of the rack by standing straight up.

2. With the bar on your upper back, take two steps back, away from the rack, and position your feet so that they are shoulder-width apart.

3. With your eyes forward, sit your butt down and back until your thighs are parallel to the floor, keeping your chest high, and your weight on your heels.

4. Straighten your legs back to the start position.

5. Complete 8–10 squats. When the set is complete, walk the bar safely back to the rack.

6. Rest and repeat for 3 sets total.

UPPER-BODY PUSH

7 | ● ■ ◆ | BENT-KNEE PUSH-UPS

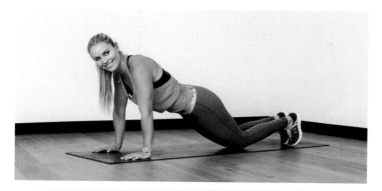

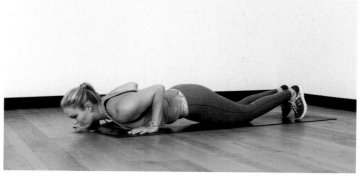

1. Kneel and place your palms flat on the floor in front of you, hands directly under shoulders.

2. Keeping your shoulders over your hands, your core tight, and your back flat, lower your chest slowly toward the floor.

3. Without letting your head drop, touch the floor with your chest, then press up through your hands to the start position.

4. Complete 12–15 push-ups.

5. Rest and repeat for 3 sets total.

UPPER-BODY PUSH

7 | ● ■ ◆ | PUSH-UPS

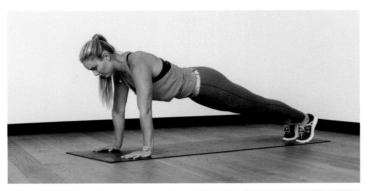

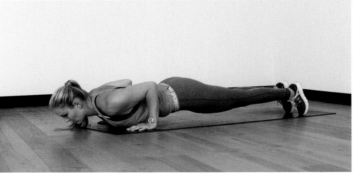

1. Position yourself facing the floor with your hands directly under your shoulders, palms pressed into the floor, arms extended straight, and toes tucked.

2. Lower your chest slowly to the floor, keeping your shoulders over your hands, core tight, back flat, and legs straight.

3. Without letting your head drop, touch the floor with your chest, then press up through your hands to the start position.

4. Complete 10–12 push-ups.

5. Rest and repeat for 3 sets total.

UPPER-BODY PUSH

7 | ● ■ ◆ | PUSH-UPS ON A HALF STABILITY BALL

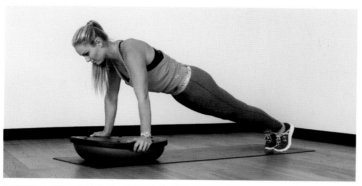

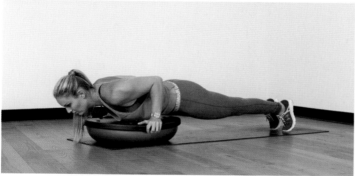

1. Flip a half stability ball over on its dome. Grip both sides of the platform so your hands are directly under your shoulders. Extend your legs straight behind you, keeping your back flat and toes tucked.

2. Lower your chest slowly to the ball, keeping your shoulders over your hands, core tight, back flat, and legs straight.

3. Without letting your head drop, try to touch the platform with your chest, then press up through your hands to the start position.

4. Complete 8–10 push-ups.

5. Rest and repeat for 3 sets total.

UPPER-BODY PUSH

8 | ● ■ ◆ | SEATED SHOULDER PRESSES

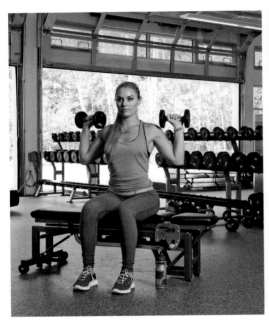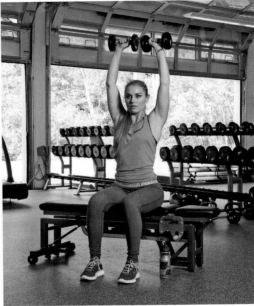

1. Sit on a bench or chair, with your chest high, shoulder blades down and back, and eyes forward. Hold a dumbbell in each hand, palms forward, and raise the weights to shoulder height.

2. Press the dumbbells straight up until your arms are extended, keeping your back flat, core tight, and eyes forward.

3. Lower the weights slowly to shoulder height.

4. Complete 12–15 presses.

5. Rest and repeat for 3 sets total.

UPPER-BODY PUSH

8 | ●■◆ | SHOULDER PRESSES ON A SWISS BALL

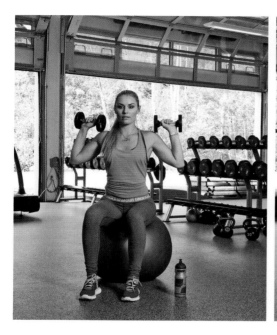 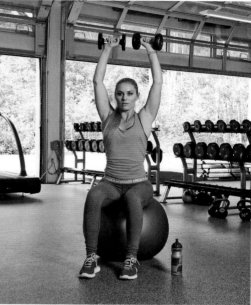

1. Sit on a Swiss ball, with your chest high, shoulder blades down and back, and eyes forward. Hold a dumbbell in each hand, palms forward, and raise the weights to shoulder height.

2. Press the dumbbells straight up until your arms are extended, keeping your back flat, core tight, and eyes forward.

3. Lower the weights slowly to shoulder height.

4. Complete 10–12 presses.

5. Rest and repeat for 3 sets total.

UPPER-BODY PUSH

8 | ●■◆ | SHOULDER PRESSES ON A SWISS BALL, LEG LIFTED

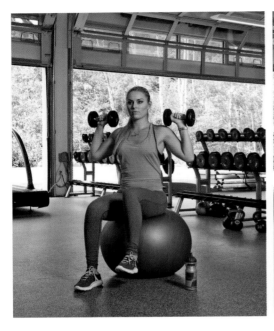 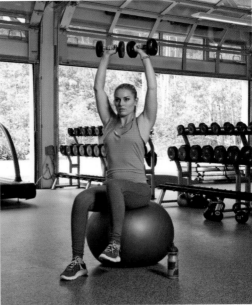

1. Sit on a Swiss ball, with your chest high, shoulder blades down and back, and eyes forward. Hold a dumbell in each hand, palms forward, and raise the weights to shoulder height. Lift your left foot slightly off the floor.

2. Press the dumbbells straight up until your arms are extended, keeping your back flat, core tight, eyes forward, and left foot lifted.

3. Lower the weights slowly to shoulder height.

4. Complete 4–5 presses with your left foot lifted, then 4–5 presses with your right lifted, for 8–10 presses total.

5. Rest and repeat for 3 sets total.

UPPER-BODY PUSH

9 | ● ■ ◆ | BENT-KNEE TRICEPS DIPS

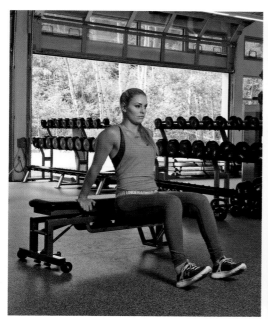 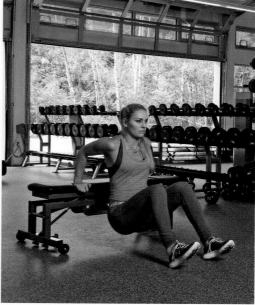

I. Sit on a chair with your hands directly under shoulders, palms down on the chair. Lift your hips off the chair until your hands support your bodyweight, keeping your knees bent.

2. Slowly lower your hips toward the floor, bending your elbows until your upper arms are parallel with the floor.

3. Raise your hips back up by straightening your arms and pressing through your hands.

4. Complete 12–15 reps.

5. Rest and repeat for 3 sets total.

UPPER-BODY PUSH

9 | ⬤ ■ ◆ | TRICEPS DIPS

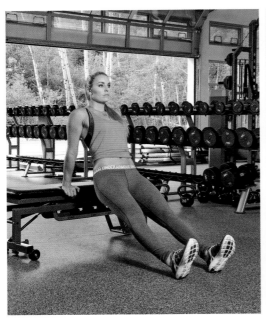 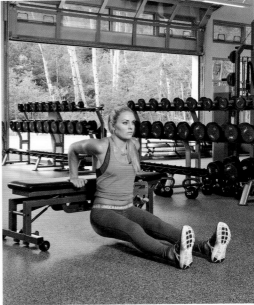

1. Sit on a chair with your hands directly under shoulders, palms down on the chair. Extend your legs in front of you, heels on the floor. Lift your hips off the chair so your hands and heels support your bodyweight, keeping your legs straight and your hips high.

2. Slowly lower your hips toward the floor, bending your elbows, keeping your legs and hips in one line, until your upper arms are parallel with the floor.

3. Raise your hips by straightening your arms and pressing through your hands.

4. Complete 10–12 reps.

5. Rest and repeat for 3 sets total.

UPPER-BODY PUSH

9 | ● ■ ◆ | BARBELL TRICEPS SKULL CRUSHERS

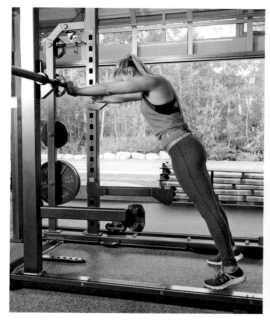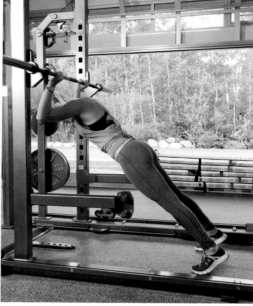

1. Place a barbell in a rack so that it is approximately the height of your sternum. With straight arms, place both hands in the middle of the bar 6–12 inches apart. Walk your feet behind you so that your body is slightly leaning forward.

2. Initiate the movement by bending your elbows and allowing your body to move toward the floor, moving your body as one unit—keeping the head, shoulders, hips, and feet in one straight line. Keep your core tight and squeeze the glutes.

3. Lower until your head moves past your hands and your temples are in line with your elbows.

4. Keeping the body in a straight line, return to the starting position by pushing your hands into the bar and squeezing your triceps.

5. Complete 8–10 reps.

6. Rest and repeat for 3 sets total.

LOWER-BODY PULL

10 | ●■◆ | SINGLE-LEG STRAIGHT LEG DEADLIFTS

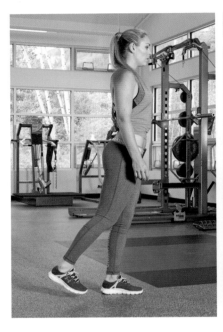 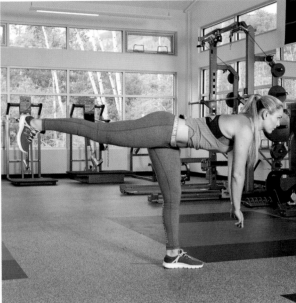

1. Stand with your feet together, toes forward, arms by your sides.

2. With a slight bend in your left knee and your back flat, bend forward by hinging from your hips while extending your right leg behind you and both arms in front of you until your right leg and back are parallel with the floor, letting your arms hang toward the floor.

3. Press your weight through your left heel to pull your leg and arms back to the start position.

4. Complete 12–15 reps standing on your left leg, then complete 12–15 reps on your right.

5. Rest and repeat for 3 sets total.

LOWER-BODY PULL

10 | ● ■ ◆ | SINGLE-LEG STRAIGHT LEG DEADLIFTS WITH A DUMBBELL

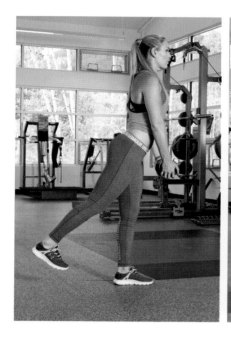 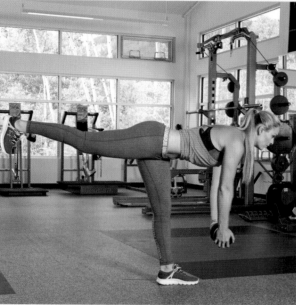

I. Stand with your feet together, toes forward, arms by your sides. Hold a dumbbell with both hands.

2. With a slight bend in your left knee and your back flat, bend forward by hinging from your hips, keeping your chest high and allowing the dumbbell to hang toward the floor, while extending your right leg behind you until your right leg and back are parallel with the floor.

3. Press your body weight through your left heel to pull your leg and the dumbbell back to the start position.

4. Complete 10–12 reps standing on your left leg, then complete 10–12 reps on your right.

5. Rest and repeat for 3 sets total.

LOWER-BODY PULL

10 | ● ■ ◆ | SINGLE-LEG STRAIGHT LEG DEADLIFTS WITH DUMBBELLS

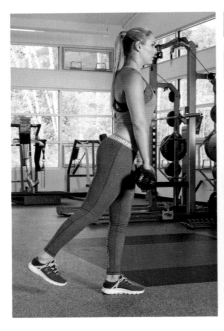 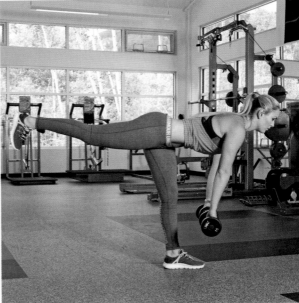

I. Perform the same exercise described in the intermediate version, but hold a dumbbell in each hand, arms by your side.

2. Allow both dumbbells to hang toward the floor as you bend forward by hinging from your hips and extending your right leg back behind you.

3. Complete 8–10 reps standing on your left leg, then complete 8–10 reps standing on your right.

4. Rest and repeat for 3 sets total.

LOWER-BODY PULL

11 | ●■◆ | DOUBLE-LEG STRAIGHT LEG DEADLIFTS WITH A DUMBBELL

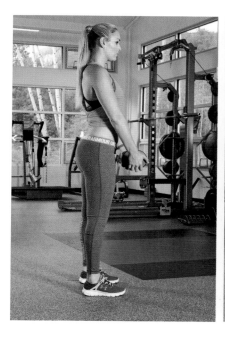 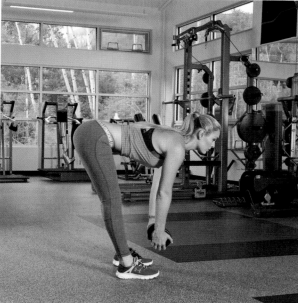

1. Stand with your feet shoulder-width apart, toes forward. Hold a light dumbbell by placing both hands under the weights, then allow the dumbbell to hang straight down toward the floor, arms extended.

2. With a slight bend in your knees, your chest high, and your shoulder blades down and back, bend forward by hinging from your hips and reaching your butt behind you as far as possible, keeping your back flat, while attempting to touch the dumbbell to the floor.

3. Straighten your legs and squeeze your glutes to return to the start position.

4. Complete 12–15 reps.

5. Rest and repeat for 3 sets total.

LOWER-BODY PULL

11 | ●■◆ | DOUBLE-LEG STRAIGHT LEG DEADLIFTS WITH A DUMBBELL

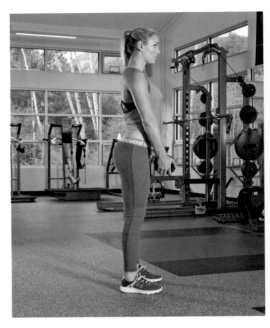 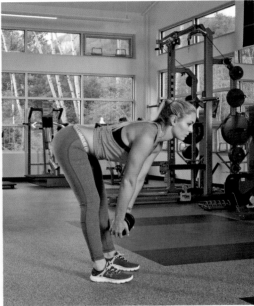

Perform the same exercise described in the beginner version but increase the weight, and complete 10–12 reps.

LOWER-BODY PULL

11 | ●■◆ | DOUBLE-LEG STRAIGHT LEG DEADLIFTS WITH DUMBBELLS

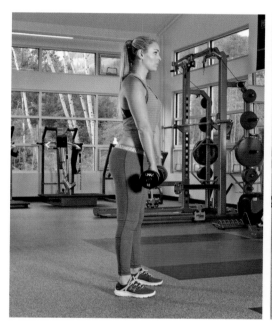 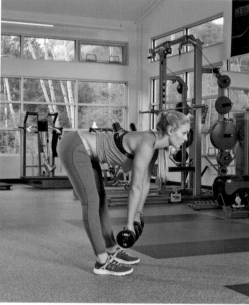

1. Stand with your feet hip-width apart, toes forward, holding a dumbbell in each hand, arms by your side.

2. With a slight bend in your knees, your chest high, and your shoulder blades down and back, bend forward by hinging from your hips, reaching your butt behind you as far as possible, allowing the dumbbells to hang straight toward the floor.

3. Bend until your upper body is parallel with the floor, keeping your chest high and your back flat.

4. Straighten your legs and squeeze your glutes to return to the start position.

5. Complete 8–10 reps.

6. Rest and repeat for 3 sets total.

LOWER-BODY PULL

12 | ● ■ ◆ | DOUBLE-LEG CURLS ON A SWISS BALL

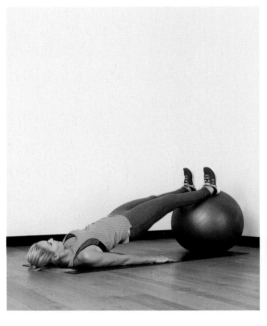 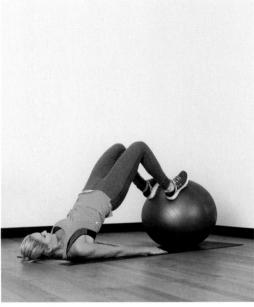

1. Lie faceup on the floor, resting your heels and ankles on a Swiss ball, arms to your sides at a 45-degree angle to your body. Lift your hips until your bodyweight rests on your upper back, keeping your core tight, back flat, and legs straight.

2. Lift your hips off the floor and use your heels to pull the ball toward you, bending your knees and squeezing your glutes, until your bodyweight rests on your shoulder blades, keeping your hips high.

3. Roll the ball back to the start position, keeping your hips off the floor.

4. Complete 12–15 curls with hips up.

5. Rest and repeat for 3 sets total.

LOWER-BODY PULL

12 ● ■ ◆ │ ECCENTRIC ALTERNATING SINGLE-LEG CURLS ON A SWISS BALL

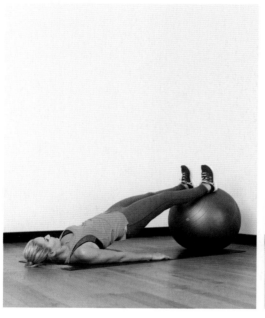 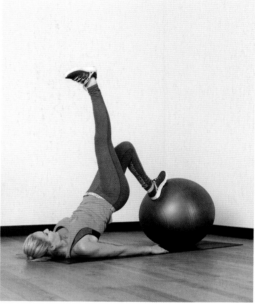

I. Start in the same position as in the beginner version.

2. Using your heels, pull the ball toward you, bending your knees and squeezing your glutes until your bodyweight rests on your shoulder blades, keeping your hips high.

3. Lift your right leg off the ball, slowly rolling the ball back to the start position with your left leg.

4. Drop your right leg to meet your left, then curl the ball back toward you with both legs before lifting your left leg off the ball and rolling back with your right.

5. Complete 10–12 curls with each leg.

6. Rest and repeat for 3 sets total.

LOWER-BODY PULL

12 | ● ■ ◆ | SINGLE-LEG CURLS ON A SWISS BALL, LEG LIFTED

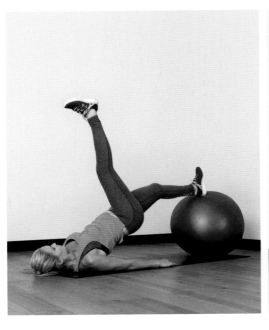 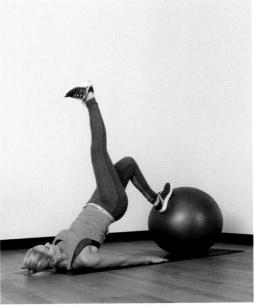

1. Start in the same position as in the beginner version, but lift your right leg off the ball before curling the ball toward you with your left leg, keeping your hips high.

2. Slowly roll the ball back to the start position, keeping your right leg lifted.

3. Curl the ball back again, with your right leg still lifted, until you've completed 8–10 curls. Lift your left leg off the ball, and complete 8–10 curls with your right.

4. Rest and repeat for 3 sets total.

UPPER-BODY PULL

13 | ●■◆ | BENT-OVER ROWS

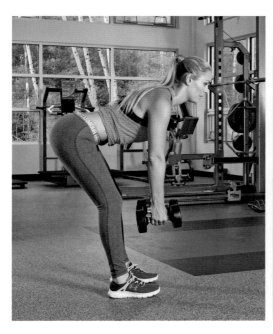 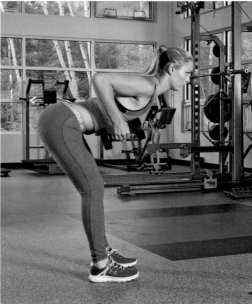

1. Stand with your toes forward, knees slightly bent. Hold a dumbbell in each hand, arms by your sides. Bend over by hinging at your hips until your upper body is parallel with the floor, keeping your chest high, your shoulder blades down, and your back flat, letting the dumbbells hang straight below your shoulders.

2. Pull the dumbbells toward you until they touch either side of your chest, squeezing your shoulder blades back and keeping your elbows close to your body.

3. Slowly lower to the start position.

4. Complete 12–15 rows.

5. Rest and repeat for 3 sets total.

UPPER-BODY PULL

13 | ●■◆ | ALTERNATE BENT-OVER ROWS

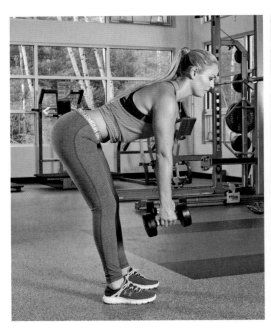 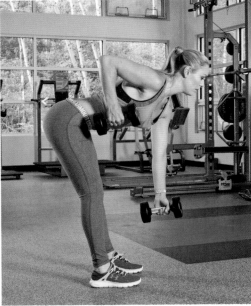

I. Stand with your toes forward, knees slightly bent. Hold a dumbbell in each hand, arms by your sides.

2. Bend over by hinging at your hips until your upper body is parallel with the floor, keeping your chest high, your shoulder blades down and back, and your back flat, letting the dumbbells hang straight below your shoulders.

3. Pull the dumbbell in your right hand toward you until it touches the right side of your chest, squeezing your shoulder blades back and keeping your elbow close to your body.

4. Lower slowly to the start position, then row up with your left arm.

5. Complete 10–12 rows with each arm.

6. Rest and repeat for 3 sets total.

UPPER-BODY PULL

13 | ●■◆ | SINGLE-ARM BENT-OVER ROWS

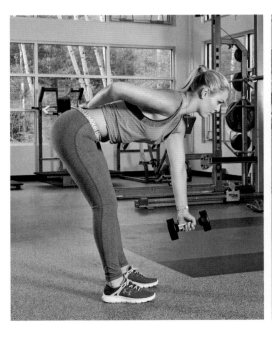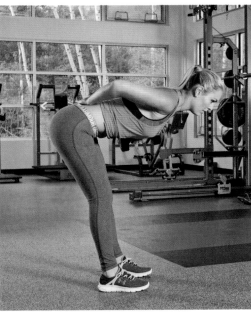

I. Stand with your toes forward, knees slightly bent. Hold only one dumbbell in your left hand and place the back of your right hand on your lower back.

2. Bend over by hinging at your hips until your upper body is parallel with the floor, keeping your chest high, your shoulder blades down and back, and your back flat, letting the dumbbell hang straight below your shoulders.

3. Pull the dumbbell toward you until it touches the left side of your chest, squeezing your shoulder blades back and keeping your elbow close to your body. Lower slowly to the start position.

4. Complete 8–10 rows on the left, then 8–10 rows on the right.

5. Rest and repeat for 3 sets total.

UPPER-BODY PULL

14 | ●■◆ | IYTs

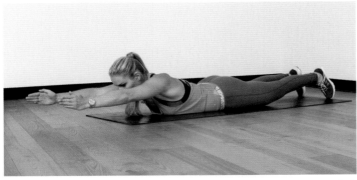

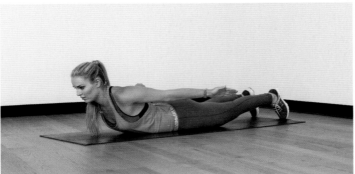

1. Lie on your stomach, chin on the floor, legs extended back, arms extended straight overhead, with your thumbs up so that your body forms the letter I.

2. Lift your arms as high as possible, using your upper back muscles and squeezing your shoulder blades back. Lower and repeat 12–15 times.

3. Move your arms to a 45-degree angle to form the letter Y. Lift your arms as high as possible, using your upper back muscles and squeezing your shoulder blades back. Lower and repeat 12–15 times.

4. Move your arms to a 90-degree angle to form the letter T. Lift your arms as high as possible, using your upper back muscles and squeezing your shoulder blades back. Lower and repeat 12–15 times.

5. Rest and repeat in all three positions for 3 sets total.

UPPER-BODY PULL

14 | ● ■ ◆ | DUMBBELL IYTs

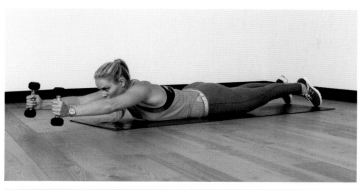

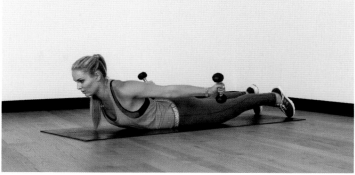

1. Start in the same position as in the beginner version, but hold a light dumbbell in each hand.

2. Perform the exercises described in the beginner version with dumbbells, except complete only 10–12 reps in each position.

3. Rest and repeat in all three positions for 3 sets total.

UPPER-BODY PULL

14 | ●■◆ | DUMBBELL IYTs ON A SWISS BALL

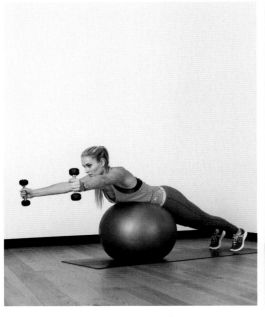 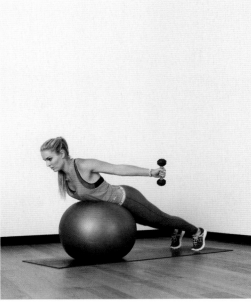

1. Rest your stomach on a Swiss ball, with your legs extended straight behind you, toes tucked. Hold a light dumbbell in each hand on either side of the ball.

2. Lift your arms in front of you until your body forms the letter I.

3. From this position, perform the exercises described in the beginner version with dumbbells, except complete only 8–10 reps in each position.

4. Rest and repeat in all three positions for 3 sets total.

UPPER-BODY PULL

15 | ● ■ ◆ | DUMBBELL PULLOVERS ON A BENCH

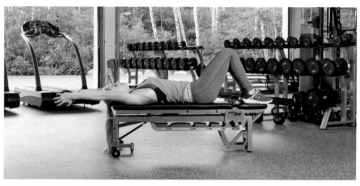

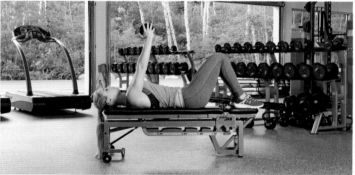

1. Lie on a bench with your knees bent and your feet flat on the bench. Hold a dumbell on either end with both hands.

2. Press the dumbbell up over your shoulders until your arms are extended.

3. With a slight bend in your elbows, stretch the dumbbell back behind your head until your forearms are parallel with the floor.

4. Keeping the slight bend in your elbows, slowly pull the dumbbell back to the start position.

5. Complete 12–15 pullovers.

6. Rest and repeat for 3 sets total.

UPPER-BODY PULL

15 | ● ■ ◆ | DUMBBELL PULLOVERS ON A BENCH

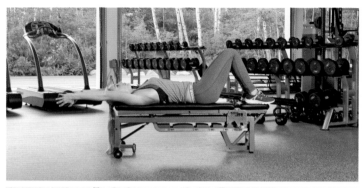

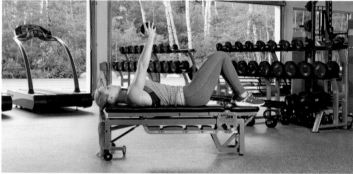

Perform the same exercise described in the beginner version but increase the weight, and complete 10–12 reps.

UPPER-BODY PULL

15 | ●■◆ | DUMBBELL PULLOVERS ON A SWISS BALL

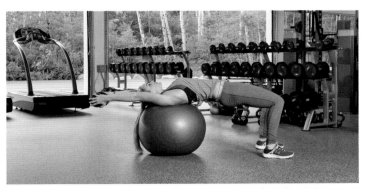

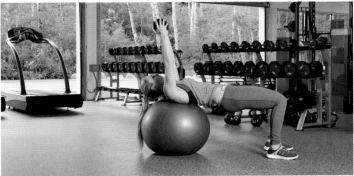

I. Rest your upper back on a Swiss ball with your knees bent and your feet flat on the floor. Hold a dumbell on either end with both hands.

2. Press the dumbbell up over your shoulders until your arms are extended.

3. With a slight bend in your elbows, stretch the dumbbell back behind your head until your forearms are parallel with the floor, keeping your hips high and your thighs parallel to the floor.

4. Keeping the slight bend in your elbows, slowly pull the dumbbell back to the start position.

5. Complete 8–10 reps.

6. Rest and repeat for 3 sets total.

CORE

16 | ●■◆ | FRONT PLANKS

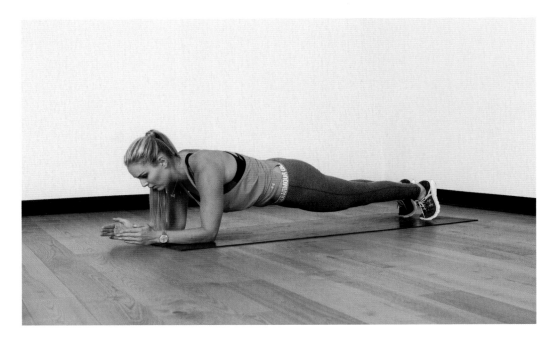

1. Lie on your stomach on the floor, with your elbows bent, forearms flat on the floor, toes tucked.

2. Press through your forearms and toes to lift your body off the floor, keeping your core tight, back flat, and legs straight so your head, back, and legs form a straight line.

3. Hold for 30 seconds before slowly lowering yourself to the start position.

4. Rest and repeat for 3 sets total.

CORE

16 | ⬤ ■ ◆ | FRONT PLANKS ON A SWISS BALL

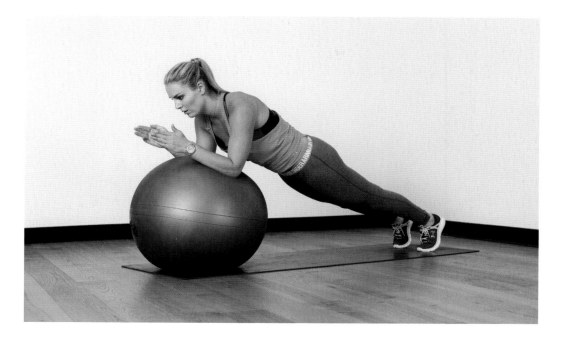

I. Rest your forearms on a Swiss ball and extend both legs directly behind you, toes tucked, so your head, shoulders, back, and legs form a straight line.

2. Hold for 30 seconds, keeping your core tight and back flat.

3. Bend your knees to the floor to release.

4. Rest and repeat for 3 sets total.

CORE

16 | ●■◆ | MOUNTAIN CLIMBERS ON A SWISS BALL

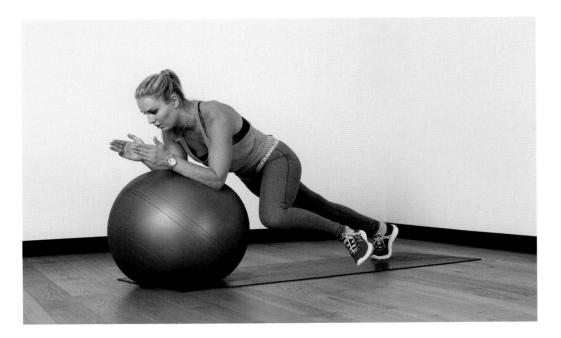

1. Rest your forearms on a Swiss ball and extend both legs directly behind you, toes tucked, so your head, shoulders, back, and legs form a straight line.

2. Bend your right knee up toward the ball, then straighten your leg and place your right foot back next to your left, keeping your back flat.

3. Then bend your left knee toward the ball, alternating legs continuously for 30 seconds, as if climbing imaginary stairs.

4. Rest and repeat for 3 sets total.

CORE

17 | ●■◆ | BENT-KNEE SIDE PLANKS

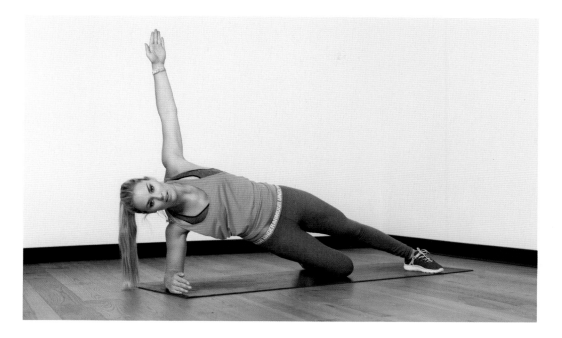

1. Lie on your right side with your right forearm flat on the floor, legs stacked, bottom knee bent, top leg straight, left hand extended in the air.

2. Lift your upper body off the floor by pressing through your right forearm until your bodyweight rests on your right forearm and right hip.

3. Then lift your hips up so your bodyweight rests only on your right forearm and knee.

4. Hold for 30 seconds, keeping your hips high.

5. Slowly lower your body, then repeat lying on your left side for 30 seconds.

6. Rest and repeat for 3 sets total on each side.

CORE

17 | ● ■ ◆ | SIDE PLANK

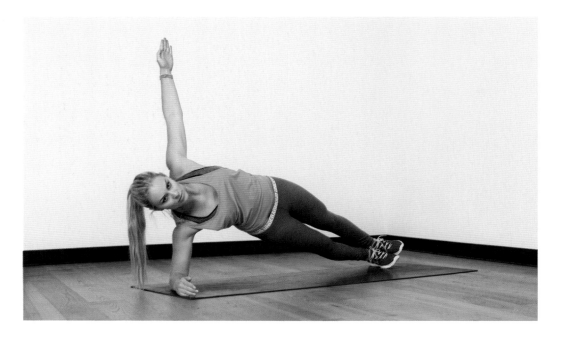

1. Lie on your right side with your right forearm flat on the floor, left hand straight up, legs extended straight.

2. Lift your entire body off the floor by pressing through your right forearm until your bodyweight rests on your right forearm and feet, and your head, back, and left hip form a straight line. Hold for 30 seconds, keeping your hips high.

3. Slowly lower your body, then repeat lying on your left side for 30 seconds.

4. Rest and repeat for 3 sets total on each side.

CORE

17 | ●■◆ | SIDE PLANK, HIP ABDUCTION

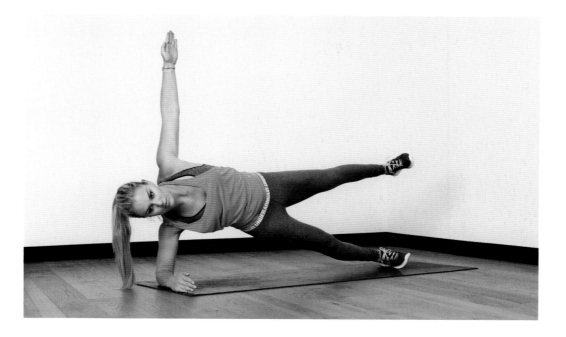

1. Lie on your right side with your right forearm flat on the floor, left hand straight up, legs extended straight.

2. Lift your entire body off the floor by pressing through your right forearm until your bodyweight rests on your right forearm and feet, and your head, back, and left hip form a straight line.

3. Lift your left leg, squeezing your left glute. Lower to meet your right leg again, and keep lifting continuously for 30 seconds, while maintaining the plank position.

4. Slowly lower your body, then repeat lying on your left side for 30 seconds.

5. Rest and repeat for 3 sets total on each side.

CORE

18 | ●■◆ | GLUTE BRIDGES

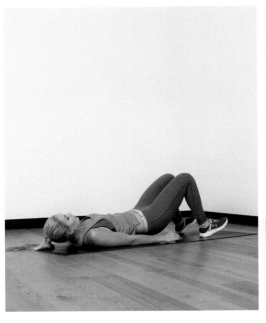
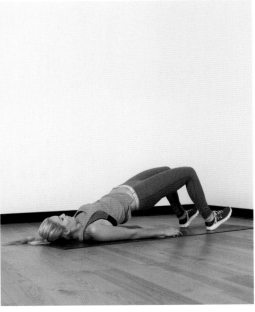

1. Lie on your back on the floor with your knees bent, your heels on the floor, arms by your sides.

2. Lift your hips by squeezing your glutes and pressing your heels into the floor, keeping your core tight and back flat, until your back and hips form a straight line.

3. Hold for 1 second, keeping your hips high, then slowly lower your hips to the floor.

4. Complete 12–15 bridges.

5. Rest and repeat for 3 sets total.

CORE

18 | ●■◆ | GLUTE BRIDGES ON A SWISS BALL

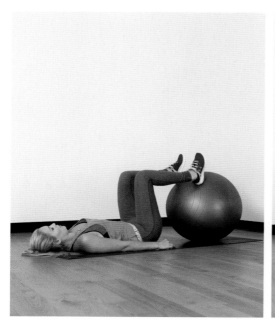 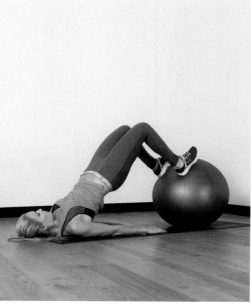

I. Lie on your back on the floor with your heels on a Swiss ball and your knees bent so your thighs are perpendicular to the floor, arms by your side.

2. Lift your hips by squeezing your glutes and pressing your heels into the ball, keeping your core tight and back flat, until your back and hips form a straight line; do not pull or push the ball.

3. Hold for I second, keeping your hips high, then slowly lower your hips to the floor.

4. Complete I0–I2 bridges.

5. Rest and repeat for 3 sets total.

CORE

18 | ● ■ ◆ | SINGLE-LEG GLUTE BRIDGES ON A SWISS BALL

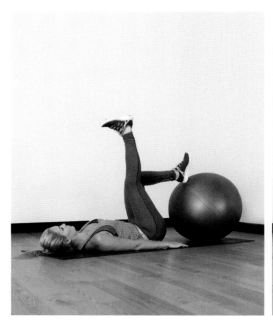 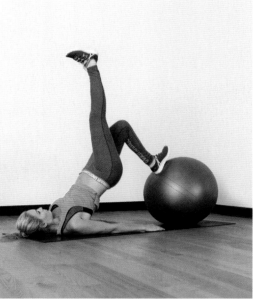

1. Lie on your back on the floor with your heels on a Swiss ball and your knees bent, arms by your side. Straighten and lift your right leg so it's perpendicular to the floor, keeping your left knee bent and your left heel on the ball.

2. Lift your hips by squeezing your glutes and pressing your left heel into the ball, keeping your core tight, back flat, and right leg extended; do not push or pull the ball.

3. Hold for 1 second, keeping your hips high, then slowly lower your hips to the floor.

4. Complete 8–10 bridges with your right leg extended, then complete 8–10 bridges with your left leg extended.

5. Rest and repeat for 3 sets total.

CORE

19 | ● ■ ◆ | **BACK EXTENSIONS**

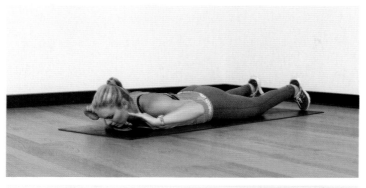

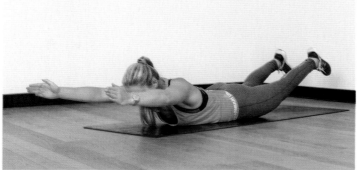

1. Lie on your stomach, chin on the floor, legs extended behind you, feet relaxed, arms by your head, thumbs up.

2. With your eyes down, extend and lift your arms and upper body and legs as high as possible, squeezing your glutes and arching your back.

3. Release slowly to the floor. Hold for 30 seconds.

4. Rest and repeat for 3 sets total.

CORE

19 | ● ■ ◆ | SUPERMANS

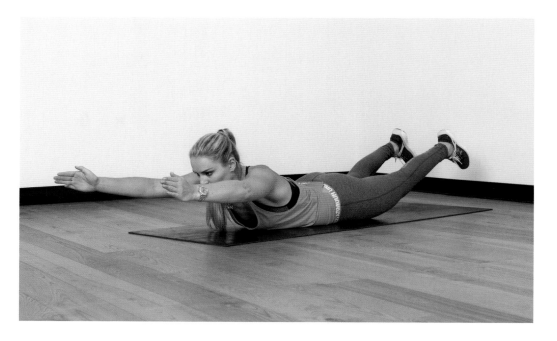

1. Lie on your stomach, chin on the floor, legs extended behind you, feet relaxed, arms extended in front of you, thumbs up.

2. With your eyes down, lift both your arms and your feet as high as possible, squeezing your glutes and arching your back.

3. Hold for 30 seconds, then release slowly to the floor.

4. Rest and repeat for 3 sets total.

CORE

19 | ●■◆ | SUPERMANS WITH DUMBBELLS

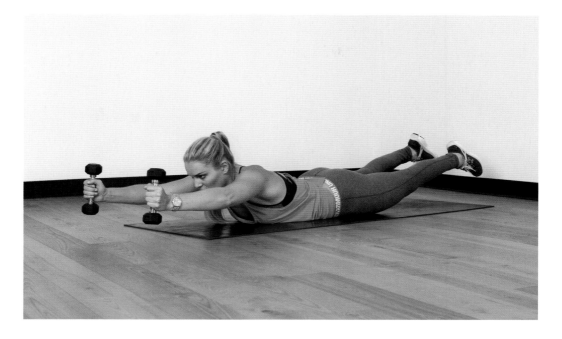

1. Perform the exercise described in the intermediate version, but hold a light dumbbell in each hand.

2. Hold the position for 30 seconds, then release slowly to the floor.

3. Rest and repeat for 3 sets total.

CORE

20 | ● ■ ◆ | BIRD DOGS

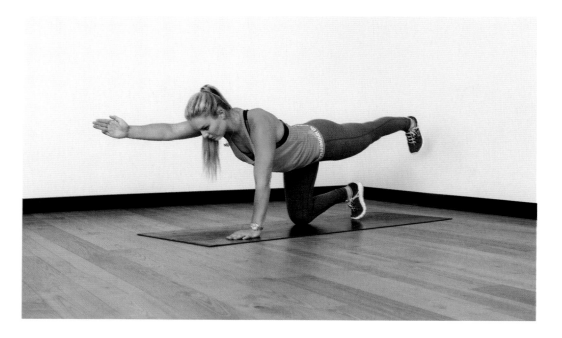

1. Kneel on your hands and knees with your hands directly under your shoulders, knees directly under your hips, eyes down, back flat, and feet relaxed.

2. Slowly extend your right arm in front of you while extending your left leg behind you, keeping your hips and shoulders square to the floor and your back flat.

3. Hold for I second, then slowly pull your arm and leg back to the start position.

4. Repeat, reaching with your left arm and right leg, alternating arms and legs until you've completed 12–15 bird dogs on either side.

5. Rest and repeat for 3 sets total.

CORE

20 | ●■◆ | **TALL PLANKS WITH ARM REACH**

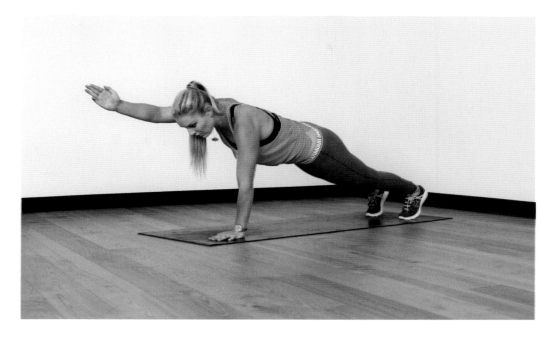

1. Start in push-up position, keeping your core tight, back flat, and legs straight so your head, back, and legs form a straight line.

2. Straighten your forearms until your arms are extended, palms pressing flat into the floor.

3. Extend your right arm directly in front of you, keeping your eyes down, core tight, hips square to the ground, and back flat.

4. Hold for I second, then lower your arm, maintaining the tall plank position.

5. Repeat, extending with your left arm, alternating arms until you've completed IO−I2 reps with each arm.

6. Rest and repeat for 3 sets total.

CORE

20 | ●■◆ | TALL PLANKS WITH ARM AND LEG REACH

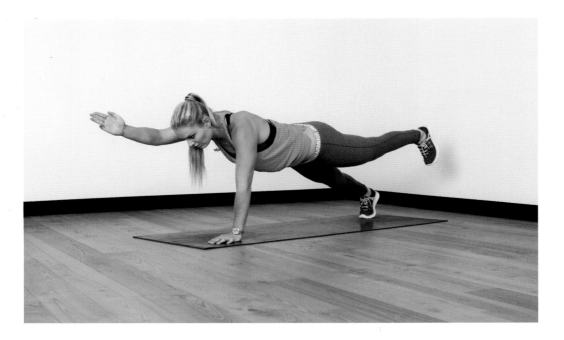

1. Start in push-up position, keeping your core tight, back flat, and legs straight so your head, back, and legs form a straight line.

2. Extend your right arm directly in front of you while lifting your left leg, keeping your eyes down, core tight, hips and shoulders square to the floor, and back flat.

3. Hold for I second, then slowly release your arm and leg, maintaining the tall plank position.

4. Repeat, extending your left arm and right leg, alternating sides until you've completed 8–I0 reps with each arm-leg combo.

5. Rest and repeat for 3 sets total.

CORE

21 | ● ■ ◆ | TRUNK TWISTS WITH WEIGHT

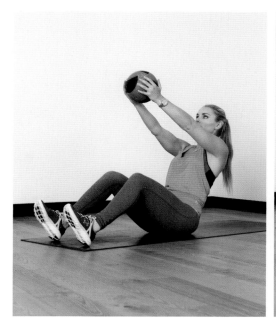 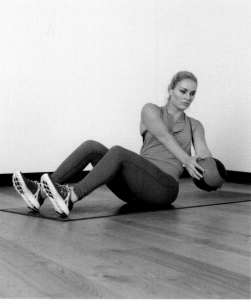

1. Sit on the floor with your knees bent, heels on the floor. Hold a medicine ball or either end of a dumbbell with both hands.

2. Stretch the weight in front of you until your arms are extended, keeping your core tight and your back flat.

3. Rotate your upper body to the left, moving the weight with you, before rotating back through your center and to your right, moving the weight with you throughout.

4. Keep rotating continuously for 12-15 reps on each side.

5. Rest and repeat for 3 sets total.

CORE

21 | ●■◆ | STANDING CHOPS

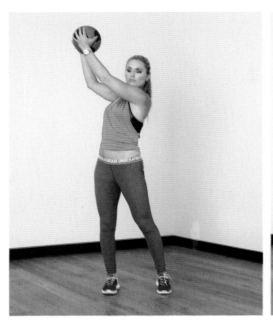 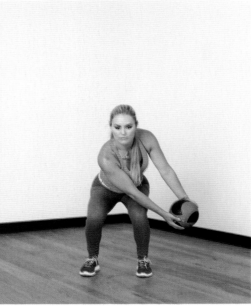

1. Stand with your feet shoulder-width apart, toes forward. Hold a medicine ball or either end of a dumbbell in both hands and lift the weight up in the air over your right shoulder.

2. Squat, moving the weight across your body until your right arm crosses your left thigh, then immediately lift it back up across your body by straightening your legs, keeping your arms extended, until the weight is above your right shoulder.

3. Immediately squat and move the weight back down to the outside of your left thigh. Keep chopping for 10–12 reps before switching to chop from your left shoulder to your right thigh.

4. Rest and repeat for 3 sets total to each side.

CORE

21 | ●■◆ | SINGLE-LEG STANDING CHOPS

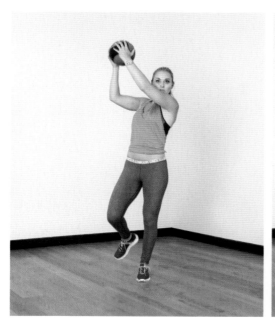 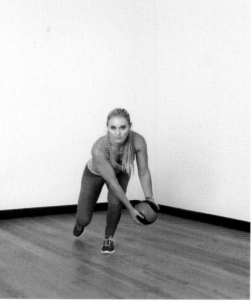

I. Perform the exercise described in the intermediate version, but stand on your left leg only, right knee bent and foot raised.

2. Chop for 8–10 reps without allowing your right foot to touch the floor before switching sides to stand on your right leg only.

3. Rest and repeat for 3 sets total to each side.

DYNAMIC STRETCHING

22 | WALKING QUAD STRETCHES

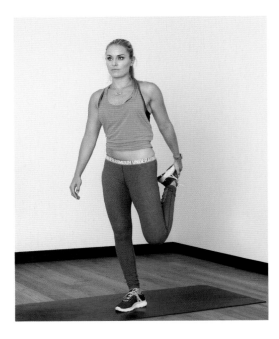

1. Stand on your right foot.

2. Kick the heel of your left foot up to your glutes, holding your foot with your left hand to stretch your left quad for a count of 2.

3. Step out of the stretch with your left foot, stepping forward onto your left leg and kicking up your right foot to stretch your right quad.

4. Keep walking and stretching until you've stretched each quad 12–15 times.

MUSCLE ACTIVATION

23 | LATERAL RESISTANCE BAND WALKS

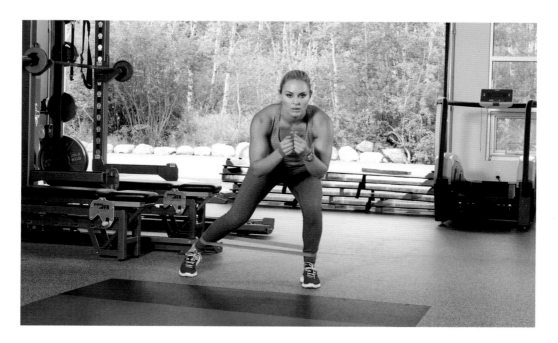

1. Place or tie a resistance band around your legs above your ankles and stand with your feet shoulder-width apart, toes forward—adjust the band until the tension is tight.

2. With a slight bend in your knees and the core tight, step sideways with your right foot, pushing against the tension, before stepping sideways to the right with your left foot, keeping your feet shoulder-width apart.

3. Keep stepping sideways to the right, one foot at a time, until you've completed 15 steps total.

4. Switch directions, stepping to the left until you've completed 15 steps total.

THE GET-STRONG CIRCUITS

Before any workout, warm up by doing 5 to 10 minutes of light aerobic activity like walking or using a Spin bike at a low resistance, followed by light foam rolling (optional), dynamic stretches like the walking quad stretch, and one to three sets of lateral resistance band walks.

 BEGINNER

CIRCUIT 1

- Split hops (p. 165)
- Split squats (p. 177)
- Seated shoulder presses (p. 186)
- Double-leg straight leg deadlifts with a dumbbell (p. 195)
- Bent-over rows (p. 201)
- Front planks (p. 210)
- Glute bridges (p. 216)

CIRCUIT 2

- Lateral line hops (p. 171)
- Side squats (p. 174)
- Bent-knee triceps dips (p. 189)
- Double-leg curls on a Swiss ball (p. 198)
- IYTs (p. 204)
- Back extensions (p. 219)
- Bent-knee side planks (p. 213)

CIRCUIT 3

- Squat jumps (p. 168)
- Squats with a dumbbell (p. 180)
- Bent-knee push-ups (p. 183)
- Single-leg straight leg deadlifts (p. 192)
- Dumbbell pullovers on a bench (p. 207)
- Bird dogs (p. 222)
- Trunk twists with weight (p. 225)

INTERMEDIATE

CIRCUIT 1

- Split squat jumps (p. 166)
- Rear-foot elevated split squats with dumbbells (p. 178)
- Shoulder presses on a Swiss ball (p. 187)
- Double-leg straight leg deadlifts with a dumbbell (p. 196)
- Alternate bent-over rows (p. 202)
- Front planks on a Swiss ball (p. 211)
- Glute bridges on a Swiss ball (p. 217)

CIRCUIT 2

- Lateral skater hops (p. 172)
- Side lunges with a dumbbell (p. 175)
- Triceps dips (p. 190)
- Eccentric alternating single-leg curls on a Swiss ball (p. 199)
- Dumbell IYTs (p. 205)
- Superman (p. 220)
- Side plank (p. 214)

CIRCUIT 3

- Tuck jumps (p. 169)
- Squats with dumbbells (p. 181)
- Push-ups (p. 184)
- Single-leg straight leg deadlifts with a dumbbell (p. 193)
- Dumbbell pullovers on a bench (p. 208)
- Tall planks with arm reach (p. 223)
- Standing chops (p. 226)

● ■ ◆ | EXPERT

CIRCUIT 1

- Scissor jumps (p. 167)
- Swiss ball rear-foot elevated split squats with dumbbells (p. 179)
- Shoulder presses on a Swiss ball, leg lifted (p. 188)
- Double-leg straight leg deadlifts with dumbbells (p. 197)
- Single-arm bent-over rows (p. 203)
- Mountain climbers on a Swiss ball (p. 212)
- Single-leg glute bridges on a Swiss ball (p. 218)

CIRCUIT 2

- Lateral skater bounds (p. 173)
- Side lunges with dumbbells (p. 176)
- Barbell triceps skull crushers (p. 191)
- Single-leg curls on a Swiss ball, leg lifted (p. 200)
- Dumbbell IYTs on a Swiss ball (p. 206)
- Superman with dumbbells (p. 221)
- Side planks, hip abduction (p. 215)

CIRCUIT 3

- Squat jumps with a dumbbell (p. 170)
- Barbell back squats (p. 182)
- Push-ups on a half stability ball (p. 185)
- Single-leg straight leg deadlifts with dumbbells (p. 194)
- Dumbbell pullovers on a Swiss ball (p. 209)
- Tall planks with arm and leg reach (p. 224)
- Single-leg standing chops (p. 227)

How to Do the Circuits

Perform one set of repetitions for the first exercise listed, then move on to the next exercise, taking as short a rest as you can comfortably between sets, until you've completed one set for all seven exercises. Repeat the circuit three times total.

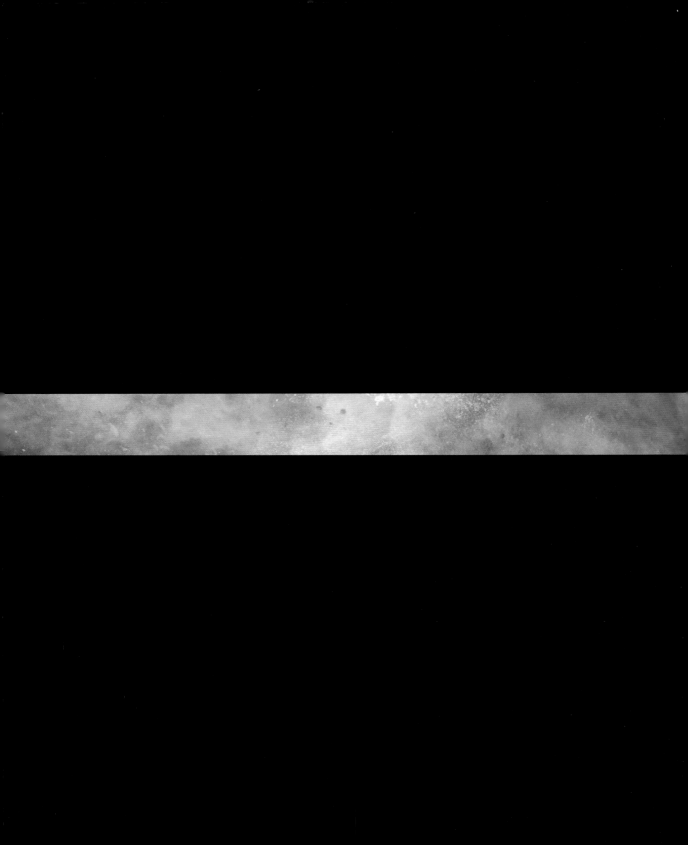

GLAM

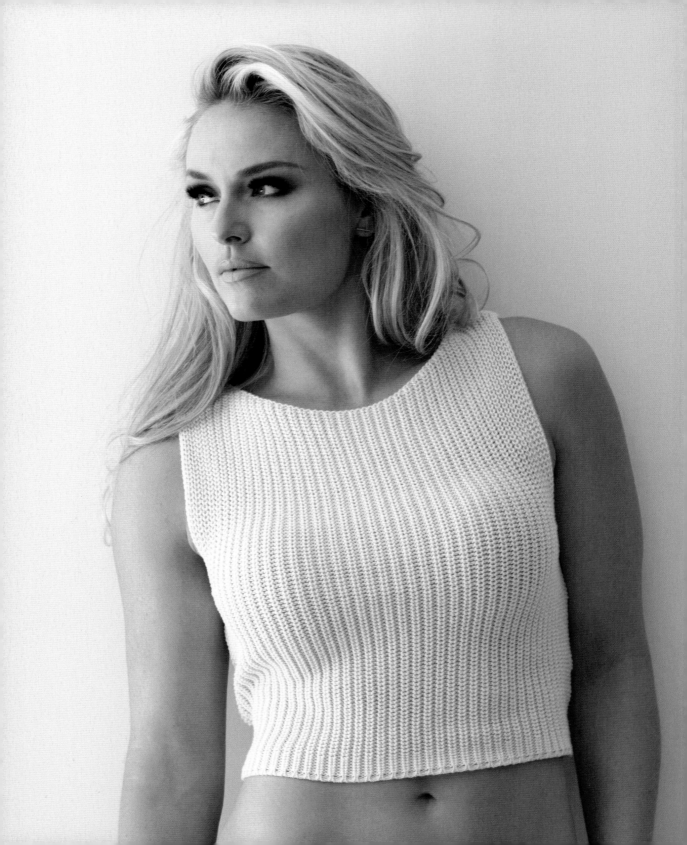

12/ LOVE YOUR BODY, CELEBRATE YOUR BEAUTY

I believe that every woman is beautiful. Every one of us has something stunning to share with the world, whether it's a special gift, an ability, an idea, or a sparkle unique in your eyes only.

The stronger you are on the inside, the more beautiful you become on the outside. To me, confidence and inner strength are the most attractive qualities a woman can possess.

I feel strong and confident when I'm working out, racing, at home in Vail with Bear and Leo, or just hanging out with my friends or family. But as is true of almost every woman, I can struggle with issues of self-assurance, especially when it comes to stereotypes surrounding physical beauty.

I love my body and how I look, and while I'm comfortable with who I am, I also know that I don't look like most models and celebrities that Hollywood and the glossy magazines promote as beautiful. Despite this, though, I'm continually subjected to other people's ideas of what beauty should be. My physical appearance is constantly analyzed by the press and public whenever I race, go on TV, attend celebrity events, get snapped by the press, pose for magazines, or even post my own pictures on social media. People talk about whether they think I've gained or lost weight; how my legs, butt, or arms look; what outfit I have on and whether it's too tight or loose-fitting; what my hair looks like; how much makeup I wear; whether I look too sexy or not sexy enough; or how my looks compare with someone else's—the judgments can feel near limitless at times.

While I've gotten pretty good at zoning out the chatter, it's still difficult not to be affected at times by what other people say—both the good stuff and the bad. And when I'm having a bad day or feeling not particularly awesome about myself for whatever reason, it can be easy to start thinking that all the other celebrities or magazine models are beautiful and that I'm not.

Sound familiar? For many women, this is a big problem: We feel like we don't fit into the conventional mold for beauty that society projects. But it's absolutely critical to realize that this mold is a projection only—what we think the image is that everyone likes—and is based on nothing in reality.

As cliché as it is, beauty is in the eye of the beholder. We have different tastes in what we consider physically attractive just as we have different tastes in food, art, music, literature, and movies. And if we all liked the same thing, how boring would the world be?

Thankfully, we don't all like the same thing, which becomes more evident when you look around the world. What's considered beautiful in Polynesia, for example, is drastically different from what's considered beautiful in Scandinavia.

Even in the United States, ideals about beauty have changed so remarkably from decade to decade that it's easy to see just how flimsy and temporal the concept of beauty can be. If you look at old films or magazines and see what people considered beautiful in the 1930s, it's much different from the standards of beauty in the forties, fifties, sixties, and later.

I've learned to be proud of how I look and to celebrate my beauty as much as I celebrate my body—because I am beautiful. And you are beautiful, too. Strength is beauty and there's beauty in strength, and the stronger you are, the more your outer and inner strength will shine through and enhance everything about you, above and below the skin.

Here are three ways I celebrate my beauty every day.

1 MAKEUP. To me, putting on makeup is like painting a canvas: The colors you choose and how you apply them is an art—and your prerogative as the artist. Whatever you choose, as long as you paint with con-

My Daily Makeup Routine

1. I always swipe my face with a makeup-removing towel, then wash with a gentle cleanser. This way, I start with a clean palette and no old makeup to mar a fresh look.

2. Before applying color, I moisturize, using a facial moisturizer with SPF so that my skin looks smooth and stays nourished and protected all day long.

3. When it comes time for color, I start with long-wear liquid eyeliner, which I apply using a thin brush to my top lash line.

4. I love neutral eye shadow, so I pick a pale palette and apply using a blending brush, with a lighter shade just below my brow area and a darker shade like brown on my eyelids.

5. On my skin, I prefer the color and feel of a concealer stick under my eyes and to cover blemishes. I use a concealer brush to apply.

6. After concealer, I lightly dust my face with foundation using a foundation brush to even my skin tone.

7. To help my eyes stand out, I use a brow pencil to fill in and define my eyebrows.

8. Contouring really completes my look, so I apply bronzer under my cheekbones and on the sides of my forehead to help accentuate the shape of my face. I also use just a touch of blush, being careful to make sure everything is blended well before going out.

9. The last thing on my face: volumizing black mascara!

viction, you'll look stunning; in other words, confidence is once again key when it comes to wearing makeup and looking good. On the other hand, those of my friends who don't wear makeup look that much more beautiful because they're doing what they want, not what society expects them to.

I love wearing makeup. While I rarely do so while I'm at home or out and about in Vail, I like to wear it when I race. It's partly psychological for me, as if I'm literally putting on a game face to compete. I also like how I look when I wear makeup, and I want to present what I feel is my best face to the world when I ski—it helps me feel more confident and powerful.

Years ago some athletes made fun of me for wearing makeup when I raced. They thought that since we were pro athletes, we weren't supposed to look pretty, too. To me, that's totally ridiculous. You don't have to choose between being athletic and being beautiful. In fact, the two go hand in hand, as most beautiful women I've met are super athletic, too.

When I'm going out to dinner or racing smaller events, I follow my daily makeup routine. But before bigger races, I am more meticulous when I apply my makeup. I like to wear more eye makeup when I ski because it makes my eyes stand out—crucial when your face is overshadowed by a big, bulbous helmet all day. Foundation and concealer also help to disguise every skier's bane—goggle tan—and bronzer keeps me from looking pale and frozen on the hill.

2 SKIN CARE. I try to pamper my skin as much as possible, especially since I live and work at altitude. I'm always outside training and racing, which takes a toll on my skin. At the same time, I like a simple regimen, as I'm often too tired from training or traveling to spend a ton of time fussing in the bathroom in the morning or at night. I wash my face with cleanser twice a day, and use a moisturizer with SPF every morning. When I feel clogged up after traveling, I'll also use an exfoliating scrub on my face. I wear plenty of skin lotion—it's dry in Vail and in the mountains—and try to reapply sunscreen to my face throughout the day. I don't care if this leaves me looking slightly pale year-round. I've learned through racing that skin cancer and premature aging are real risks, no matter your age, especially if you spend a lot of time outdoors.

3 HAIR. I'm proud of my hair. It's long, thick, and healthy—and all of it's mine. When I started attending more red-carpet events, I was surprised to learn how many women wear extensions to make their hair look thicker, longer, or fuller. I'm thankful for good hair genes, but I also know that I have healthy hair because I eat a balanced diet of real food with enough calories, fat, and other nutrients to help it thicken and grow.

I have to wash my hair daily because I work out every day, which makes it dry, so I use a moisturizing hair mask twice a week. Spray-on heat protector is also a must whenever I blow-dry my hair to prevent it from drying out even more.

All in all, it takes me no more than ten minutes to get ready in the morning—a good thing because I often have to wake up early to work out, race, or travel. But I also know some women who like to take their time getting ready; for them, a leisurely and luxurious routine makes them feel good about themselves and helps them better celebrate their beauty and body. Similar to eating and exercising, it's all about finding what makes you feel the best, because ultimately, when you feel your best, you look your best.

My Daily Skin-Care Routine

1. Whether I'm in the shower or at my bathroom sink, I always start by washing my face with a gentle cleanser.

2. If I'm traveling, I'll also exfoliate using a light scrub to help my skin look fresh and revived.

3. Because my skin can be very dry, I'm vigilant about applying moisturizer right after I wash my face or shower, before the water can evaporate and further dry out my skin. I always use a facial moisturizer with SPF and an unscented lotion for my body that won't conflict with my perfume.

4. My skin-care regimen doesn't change if I'm racing or before a big event. I've found that daily cleansing and moisturizing is key to helping my skin stay as nourished and healthy as possible.

My Daily Hair Routine

1. I shampoo every day because I work out every day. I also apply a heavy moisturizing conditioner every time I shampoo, since my hair gets dry, especially in the winter and at higher altitudes.

2. Twice a week, I use a deep moisturizing mask in lieu of conditioner and leave it on for at least ten or more minutes. This helps my hair stay healthy, soft, and full.

3. If I'm going out, I'll blow-dry my hair after misting on some heat-protecting spray first to keep it from drying out further. But if I don't have any plans, I'll let my hair air-dry so that it stays healthier over time.

4. When I want to style my hair, I use a round brush while blow-drying, which helps add volume, shape, and smoothness. I'm not very adept at using a curling iron, so I'll usually wear my hair straight unless a professional styles it.

5. I don't like hair spray or gel, so once I'm done styling, I'm ready to go, au naturel!

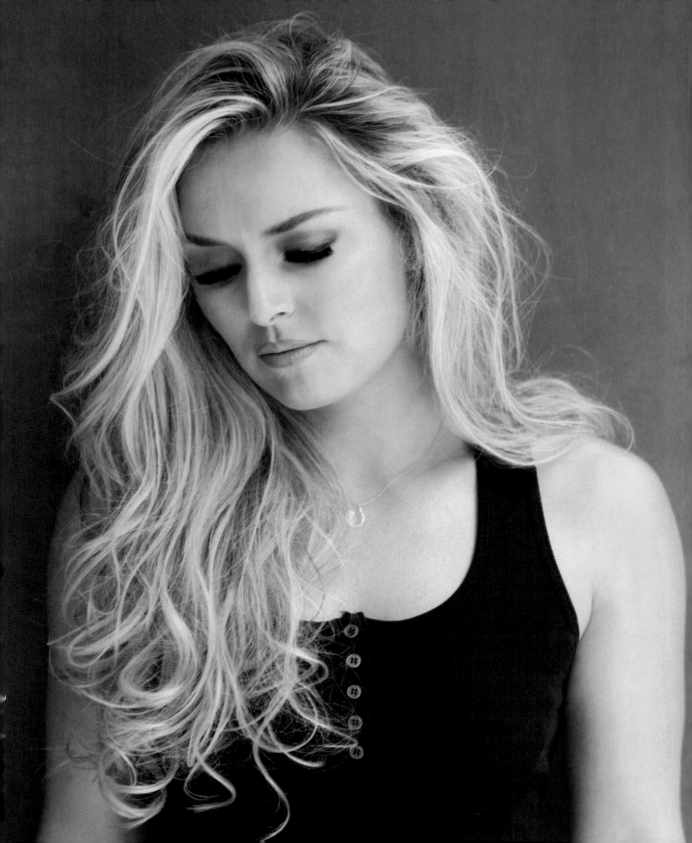

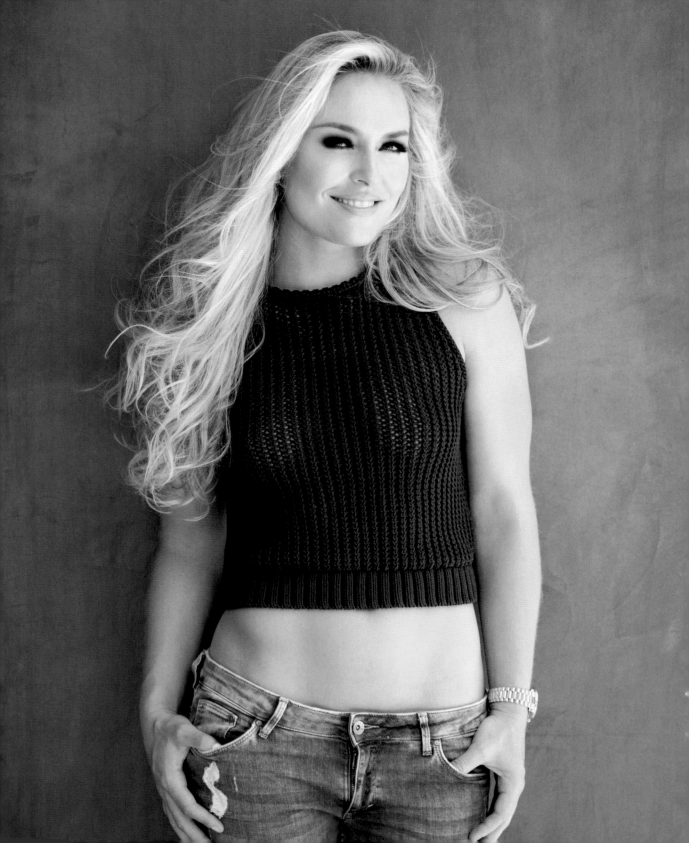

ACKNOWLEDGMENTS

I'd like to thank my family who sacrificed so much to get me to this point. I would not be in a position to even write a book if not for you. Thanks to all of my coaches and trainers along the way who helped guide and shape me both personally and professionally, and who helped pick me up after injuries so that I could break records. To all of my friends who have stood by me even when I leave the country for months at a time and never answer my phone, thank you for still standing by me! And to everyone who helped make this book possible. My team: Mark Ervin, Sue Dorf, Lewis Kay, Carly Morgan, and Jay Mandel. From William Morrow: Lisa Sharkey, Amy Bendell, Alieza Schvimer, Daniella Valladares, Lynn Grady, Michael Barrs, Kendra Newton, Mary Ann Petyak, Shelby Meizlik, Heidi Richter, Ashley Tucker, and Serena Wang. Everyone who helped on our amazing photo shoots: Alexander Bunt, Lindsay Winninger, Lauren Ross, Madison Guest, Charles Strahan, Karan Mitchell, Jesse Starr Photography, Minturn Fitness Center, Tori Hanna, and Vanessa Cella. This project was no small task and took a lot of effort on many people's parts, so thank you!

"I've learned to be proud of how I look and to celebrate my beauty as much as I celebrate my body— because I am beautiful. And you are beautiful, too. Strength is beauty and there's beauty in strength."